DASH DIET

THE COMPLETE GUIDE

IMPROVE YOUR HEALTH WITH A LOW-SODIOUM DIET

130 Delicious Recipes, 30-Day Diet Meal Plan, All Tips for Success

Author: OLIVER GART

DASH DIET PLAN

TABLE OF CONTENTS

CHAPTER ONE 22

ABOUT DASH DIET 22

DASH DIET DEFINITION 23

MORE ON DASH DIET 25

DASH DIET STARTUP 27

EFFECT OF DASH DIET 29

HABIT CHECKLIST OF DASH DIET 31

DOS AND CONS OF THE DASH DIET 33

CHAPTER TWO 34

FEATURES OF DASH DIET 34

TYPES OF DASH DIET 34

DASH DIET LAWS 35

ADVANTAGES OF FOLLOWING THE DASH DIET 36

DISADVANTAGES OF DASH DIET 37

DASH DIET BELIEVERS 38

IS DASH DIET FOR ALL 39

CHAPTER THREE 41

THE SODIUM EFFECT 41

SODIUM PHRASES AND MEANING 41

THE SODIUM PROBLEM 42

SODIUM DEFICIENCY 44

SODIUM-RICH PRODUCTS NOT RECOMMENDED ON A DASH DIET: 46

HOW TO REDUCE SODIUM 47

CHAPTER FOUR 49

DASH FOOD INTAKE 49

GOOD FOOD FOR DIET DASH 49

AVOIDABLE FOOD FOR DIET DASH 51

DASH DIET IN ACTION 51

TIPS TO START WITH DASH DIET 52

STRATEGIES FOR DEALING WITH THE DASH DIET 53

SUCCESS TIPS ON DASH DIET 54

CHAPTER FIVE 56

ABOUT HYPERTENSION 56

EFFECT ON ARTERIAL HYPERTENSION 57

DASH DIET FOR HIGH BLOOD PRESSURE 58

IMPACT OF THE DASH DIET ACCORDING TO BASELINE BLOOD PRESSURE 64

RULES TO FOLLOW 66

DASH AND WEIGHT LOSS 67

HOW TO LOSE WEIGHT WITH THE DASH DIET 68

WHAT TO DO IF YOU CAN'T LOSE WEIGHT 71

DASH DIET AND PHYSICAL EXERCISE 71

DASH DIET EXERCISES 73

CHAPTER SIX 77

DASH DIET PROCESS 77

DASH DIET SHOPPING 77

STARTING A DASH DIET 82

WORKABILITY OF DASH DIET 83

COOKING FOR DASH DIET 83

HANDLING BARRIERS AND SLIDES IN DASH DIET 85

CHAPTER SEVEN 87

DASH - MENU AND ITS COMPOSITION 87

30 DAYS DASH MEAL PLAN 92

DAY 1 92
BREAKFAST: EGG TOAST WITH SALSA — 92
LUNCH: SMOKED SALMON PITA BREAD, EGG CREAM AND GORGONZOLA CHEESE WITH PISTACHIO TOPPING — 93
DINNER: BAKED SEA BASS WITH STEAMED VEGETABLES. — 94

DAY 2 96
BREAKFAST: CHICKEN BREAST SANDWICH — 96
DINNER: BRUSSELS SPROUTS SOUP WITH MUSHROOMS — 97

DAY 3 99
BREAKFAST: PECAN PIE RECIPE — 99
LUNCH: SPINACH SALAD RECIPE — 100
DINNER: CHICKEN WITH ORZO SALAD — 101

DAY 4 103
MORNING: PUMPERNICKEL WITH LETTUCE, HARZ CHEESE AND APPLE — 103
LUNCH: TARRAGON TURKEY WITH MANGETOUT AND WILD RICE — 104
DINNER: GREEN-YELLOW BEAN SALAD WITH RED ONIONS — 105

DAY 5 107
BREAKFAST: FIG & HONEY YOGURT — 107
LUNCH: SALAD WITH WHITE BEANS, EGG AND CROUTONS — 107
DINNER: SALAD WITH RED RICE — 109

DAY 6 111
BREAKFAST: YOGURT WITH NUTS & RASPBERRIES — 111
LUNCH: ROASTED PEPPER ROLLS — 112
DINNER: HUMMUS OF CECI WITH SWEET POTATO SLICES — 112

DAY 7 114
BREAKFAST: PEANUT-BUTTER CINNAMON TOAST — 114
LUNCH: PITA WITH GRILLED TURKEY MEATBALLS — 115
DINNER: LEMON-HERB SALMON WITH CAPONATA & FARRO — 116

DAY 8 119

BREAKFAST: VEGETARIAN SPAGHETTI SAUCE	119
LUNCH: SPINACH SALAD RECIPE	120
DINNER: CHICKPEAS WITH SPINACH, RAISINS AND PINE NUTS	120

DAY 9 123
BREAKFAST: TUNA SALAD SANDWICH RECIPE	123
LUNCH: SPINACH ARTICHOKE DIP	124
DINNER: ZUCCHINI LASAGNA RECIPE	125

DAY 10 129
BREAKFAST: APPLE SALAD WITH FGS AND ALMONDS	129
LUNCH: CARAMELIZED BALSAMIC VINAIGRETTE	130
DINNER: RICH CHICKEN SALAD RECIPE	130

DAY 11 133
BREAKFAST: SAUTEED BANANAS WITH CINNAMON	133
LUNCH: HAM AND CHEESE SANDWICH	134
DINNER: CHICKEN AND SPANISH RICE RECIPE	135

DAY 12 137
BREAKFAST: HOMEMADE ALMOND AND APPLE GRANOLA	137
LUNCH: AVOCADO SALSA	138
DINNER: PORK SLICE WITH PEAR MAPLE SAUCE	139

DAY 13 141
BREAKFAST: TEMPERED QUINOA AND SMOKED TOFU SALAD	141
LUNCH: VEAL FILLET MEDALLION WITH SHERRY AND MUSHROOM SAUCE	143
DINNER: SPICY BAKED FISH	144

DAY 14 146
BREAKFAST: VINAIGRETTE SALADS	146
LUNCH: ITALIAN GREEN BEANS AND CHEESE WITH PENNE SALAD	147
DINNER: QUESADILLAS WITH SMOKED SHRIMP	148

DAY 15 150
BREAKFAST: GOLDEN BROWN GRANOLA RECIPE	150
LUNCH: CHICKPEA AND PEANUT BUTTER HUMMUS	151
DINNER: THE GREEN SALAD WITH EGGS AND CUCUMBERS	152

DAY 16 154
- BREAKFAST: TUNA SALAD RECIPE — 154
- LUNCH: CITRUS VINAIGRETTE — 155
- DINNER: FAJITAS CHICKEN FRY — 156

DAY 17 157
- BREAKFAST: DELI YOGURT WITH STRAWBERRIES — 157
- LUNCH: ARTICHOKE SALAD — 158
- DINNER: THAI LONG GRILLED RECIPE — 160

DAY 18 162
- BREAKFAST: LENTIL AND GREEK FETA SALAD — 162
- LUNCH: MAPLE OATMEAL WITH PRUNES AND PLUMS — 163
- DINNER: MINTED ENDIVE AND POTATOES RECIPE — 164

DAY 19 166
- BREAKFAST: COOL SPICY ORANGE AND CUCUMBER SALAD — 166
- LUNCH: SPICY BLACK BEAN CORN SOUP — 167
- DINNER: MEXICAN CHICKEN WITH OLIVES AND RAISINS RECIPE — 169

DAY 20 171
- BREAKFAST: SUNRISE BLUEBERRY PANCAKES RECIPE — 171
- LUNCH: PINEAPPLE AND CHOPS WITH CHILI SLAW — 172
- DINNER: CHICKEN AND TOFU STIR FRY — 173

DAY 21 175
- BREAKFAST: BERRIES YOGURT POPS RECIPE — 175
- LUNCH: SICILIAN SPAG AND TUNA RECIPE — 175
- DINNER: CURRIED PORK TENDERLOIN IN APPLE CIDER — 177

DAY 22 179
- BREAKFAST: RASPBERRY CHOCOLATE SCONES — 179
- LUNCH: BEAN AND CORN SALAD — 180
- DINNER: SCRAMBLED POTATOES AND MEAT — 181

DAY 23 183
- BREAKFAST: BANANA FRITTERS WITH OATMEAL — 183
- LUNCH: TWO-BEAN MANGO SALAD — 183

DINNER: BORDATINO WITH BEANS, BLACK CABBAGE AND CORN ... 184

DAY 24 ... 186
BREAKFAST: CHICKPEA POLENTA WITH OLIVES ... 186
LUNCH: SOBA WITH BROCCOLI AND MUSHROOMS ... 187
DINNER: COCONUT SHRIMP ... 189

DAY 25 ... 191
BREAKFAST: BUCKWHEAT PANCAKES ... 191
LUNCH: FRESH TOMATO CROSTINI ... 192
DINNER: BAKED APPLES WITH CHERRIES AND ALMOND ... 193

DAY 26 ... 195
BREAKFAST: ALMOND AND APRICOT BISCOTTI ... 195
LUNCH: APPLE DUMPINGS ... 195
DINNER: BASIL PESTO STUFFED MUSHROOM ... 197

DAY 27 ... 199
BREAKFAST: RASPBERRY CRANBERRY SPINACH SALAD ... 199
LUNCH: TOMATO SALAD WITH AVOCADO CUBES ... 199
DINNER: SCRAMBLED EGGS WITH ASPARAGUS ... 201

DAY 28 ... 202
BREAKFAST: FAT-FREE YOGURT DRESSING RECIPE ... 202
LUNCH: CRISPY POTATO SKINS ... 203
DINNER: SCALLION RICE ... 204

DAY 29 ... 206
BREAKFAST: JICAMA & MANGO SALAD ... 206
LUNCH: PUMPKIN CREAM CHEESE DIP OR SPREAD ... 206
DINNER: RICE AND BAKED CHICKEN WITH ONION AND TARRAGON ... 208

DAY 30 ... 210
BREAKFAST: SALMON WITH SOY AND GINGER ... 210
LUNCH: ASPARAGUS AND CHICKEN BREAST PENNETTE ... 211
DINNER: BRUSSELS SPROUTS AND TOASTED ALMONDS ... 211

CONCLUSION ... 214

DASH DIET COOKBOOK

TABLE OF CONTENTS

INTRODUCTION 218

CHAPTER ONE 223

MAIN DISH RECIPE 223

TARRAGON TURKEY WITH MANGETOUT AND WILD RICE 223

CHICKEN WITH ORZO SALAD 225

GLAZED TURKEY BREAST WITH FRUIT STUFFING 227

CHICKEN SALAD WITH ORANGES AND BLACK OLIVES 228

POLENTA WITH CHICKEN AND VEGETABLE SAUCE 229

ITALIAN GREEN BEANS AND CHEESE WITH PENNE SALAD 230

GREEN-YELLOW BEAN SALAD WITH RED ONIONS 231

LEMON-HERB SALMON WITH CAPONATA & FARRO 233

CHICKPEAS WITH SPINACH, RAISINS AND PINE NUTS 235

HUMMUS OF CECI WITH SWEET POTATO SLICES 237

AVOCADO CREAM AND CANNELLINI BEANS FLAVORED WITH LIME 239

SPINACH SALAD RECIPE 240

PITA WITH GRILLED TURKEY MEATBALLS 242

CHICKPEA POLENTA WITH OLIVES 244

CHAPTER TWO 246

SNACKS RECIPES 246

STRAWBERRY FROZEN YOGURT SQUARES 246

WHOLE WHEAT MUFFINS 248

LIGHTENED-UP PEANUT DIPPING SAUCE 250

ZUCCHINI WALNUT MUFFINS 252

LOW FAT PUMPKIN BREAD 254

TWO TOMATO BRUSCHETTA 256

PUMPKIN CHAI SMOOTHIE 258

PUMPKIN PIE SPICED YOGURT 259

POPEYE POWER SMOOTHIE 260

SKILLET GRANOLA 261

CHAPTER THREE 262

SIDE DISHES RECIPE 262

CAULIFLOWER WITH POTATOES 262

APPLE GRANOLA WITH NO ADDED SUGAR 263

FRIED GREEN BEANS WITH PARMESAN 264

ROASTED BUTTERNUT SQUASH FRIES 265

ROAST CHICKEN WITH POTATOES AND FRIED PLANTAINS 266

GRILLED PINEAPPLE 267

PUMPKIN CREAM CHEESE DIP OR SPREAD 268

LEMON CHEESECAKE 269

CHAPTER FOUR 270

BEVERAGE RECIPE 270

STRAWBERRY SMOOTHIE 270

MINTY LIME ICED TEA 271

OATMEAL WITH MILK AND CINNAMON 272

BANANA AND ORANGE JUICE SMOOTIE 273

WATER MELON CRANBERRY AGUA FRESCA 274

CHAPTER FIVE 275

SALAD RECIPE 275

CUCUMBER PINEAPPLE SALAD 275

GULAS AND AVOCADO SALAD WITH GINGER AND LIME VINAIGRETTE 276

DILLED SHRIMP SALAD ON LETTUS LEAVES 278

POTATO SALAD 279

GREEN SALAD WITH CHAYOTE AND PUMPKIN 280

GOJI BERRY SALAD WITH TANGERINE AND SPINACH 281

CHAPTER SIX 282

SANDWISH RECIPE 282

TUNA SALAD SANDWICHES 282

TURKEY WRAPS 283

BUFFALO CHICKEN SALAD WRAPS 284

CHICKEN SLIDERS 285

CHICKEN BURRITOS 286

CHAPTER SEVEN 287

SOUP RECIPE 287

CARROT SOUP 287

MUSHROOM AND PEARL BARLEY SOUP 288

LOW SODIUM GRILLED CHICKEN 289

CURRIED CREAM OF TOMATO SOUP WITH APPLES 290

VEGETRIAN CHILI 291

ROASTED PUMPKIN SOUP 293

CHAPTER EIGHT 295

BREAKFAST RECIPES 295

BANANA FRITTERS WITH OATMEAL 295

ALMOND AND APRICOT BISCOTTI 296

FAT FREE YOGURT DRESSING RECIPE 297

SALMON WITH SOY AND GINGER 299

LENTIL AND GREEK FETA SALAD 300

TEMPERED QUINOA AND SMOKED TOFU SALAD 302

HOMEMADE ALMOND AND APPLE GRANOLA 304

DELI YOGURT WITH STRAWBERRIES 306

BERRIES YOGURT POPS RECIPE 308

PEANUT-BUTTER CINNAMON TOAST 309

RASPBERYY CRANBERRY SPINASH SALAD 311

BUCKWHEAT PANCAKES 312

SUNRISE BLUE BERRY PANCAKES RECIPE 314

COOL SPICY ORANGE AND CUCUMBER SALAD 316

JICAMA & MANGO SALAD 318

EGG TOAST WITH SALSA 319

RASPBERRY CHOCOLATE SCONES 321

SAUTEED BANANAS WITH CINNAMON 323

VINAIGRETTE SALADS 324

PECAN PIE RECIPE 326

TUNA SALAD SANDWICH RECIPE 328

FIG & HONEY YOGURT	330
GOLDEN BROWN GRANOLA	331
APPLE SALAD WITH FGS AND ALMONDS	333
YOGURT WITH NUTS & RASPBERRIES	335
PUMPERNICKEL WITH LETTUCE, HARZ CHEESE AND APPLE	337
CHICKEN BREAST SANDWICH	339
TUNA SALAD RECIPE	341
VEGETARIAN SPAGHETTI SAUCE	343
CHAPTER NINE	345
LUNCH RECIPES	345
SOBA WITH BROCCOLI AND MUSHROOMS	345
PUMPKIN CREAM CHEESE DIP OR SPREAD	348
CITRUS VINAIGRETTE	350
CRISPY POTATO SKINS	351
FRESH TOMATO CROSTINI	353
APPLE DUMPINGS	355
ARTICHOKE SALAD	357
PINEAPPLE AND CHOPS WITH CHILI SLAW	359
SPICY BLACK BEAN CORN SOUP	361
ASPARAGUS AND CHICKEN BREAST PENNETTE	364

TWO-BEAN MANGO SALAD 366

TOMATO SALAD WITH AVOCADO CUBES... 367

SICILIAN SPAG AND TUNA RECIPE 369

SPINACH ARTICHOKE DIP 371

VEAL FILLET MEDALLION WITH SHERRY AND MUSHROOM SAUCE 373

MAPLE OATMEAL WITH PRUNES AND PLUMS 375

ROASTED PEPPER ROLLS 376

CARAMELIZED BALSAMIC VINAIGRETTE 377

HAM AND CHEESE SANDWICH 379

BEAN AND CORN SALAD 381

SMOKED SALMON PITA BREAD, EGG CREAM AND GORGONZOLA CHEESE WITH PISTACHIO TOPPING 383

CHICKPEA AND PEANUT BUTTER HUMMUS 385

AVOCADO SALSA 387

SALAD WITH WHITE BEANS, EGG AND CROUTONS 389

CHAPTER TEN 391

DINNER RECIPES 391

BRUSSELS SPROUTS AND TOASTED ALMONDS 391

SCRAMBLED EGGS WITH ASPARAGUS 393

BASIL PESTO STUFFED MUSHROOM 394

- RICE AND BAKED CHICKEN WITH ONION AND TARRAGON 396
- SCRAMBLED POTATOES AND MEAT 398
- ZUCCHINI LASAGNA RECIPE 399
- SCALLION RICE 402
- BORDATINO WITH BEANS, BLACK CABBAGE AND CORN 404
- MINTED ENDIVE AND POTATOES RECIEPE 406
- MEXICAN CHICKEN WITH OLIVES AND RAISINS RECIPE 408
- SPICY BAKED FISH 410
- BAKED APPLES WITH CHERRIES AND ALMOND 412
- CURRIED PORK TENDERLOIN IN APPLE CIDER 413
- COCONUT SHRIMP 415
- THAI LONG GRILLED RECIPE 417
- RICH CHICKEN SALAD RECIPE 419
- CHICKEN AND TOFU STIR FRY 421
- QUESADILLAS WITH SMOKED SHRIMP 423
- CHICKEN AND SPANISH RICE RECIPE 425
- THE GREEN SALAD WITH EGGS AND CUCUMBERS 427
- FAJITAS CHICKEN FRY 429
- PORK SLICE WITH PEAR MAPLE SAUCE 430
- SALAD WITH RED RICE 432

BRUSSELS SPROUTS SOUP WITH MUSHROOMS 434

BAKED SEA BASS WITH STEAMED VEGETABLES 436

FREQUENTLY ASKED QUESTIONS 438

CONCLUSION 444

DASH DIET PLAN

Learn To Eat Well.
You Lose Weight, Cholesterol Decreases and Blood Pressure Returns to Normal.

Author: OLIVER GART

© **Copyright 2020 by Oliver Gart - All rights reserved.**

The content contained within this book may not be reproduced, duplicated or transmitted without direct written permission from the author or the publisher.
Under no circumstances will any blame or legal responsibility be held against the publisher, or author, for any damages, reparation, or monetary loss due to the information contained within this book. Either directly or indirectly

Legal Notice:
This book is copyright protected. This book is only for personal use. You cannot amend, distribute, sell, use, quote or paraphrase any part, or the content within this book, without the consent of the author or publisher.

Disclaimer Notice:
Please note the information contained within this document is for educational and entertainment purposes only. All effort has been executed to present accurate, up to date, and reliable, complete information. No warranties of any kind are declared or implied. Readers acknowledge that the author is not engaging in the rendering of legal, financial, medical or professional advice. The content within this book has been derived from various sources. Please consult a licensed professional before attempting any techniques outlined in this book.

By reading this document, the reader agrees that under no circumstances is the author responsible for any losses, direct or indirect, which are incurred as a result of the use of information contained within this document, including, but not limited to, — errors, omissions, or inaccuracies.

INTRODUCTION

Dash Diet's diet plan is aimed at removing salt and fat for a healthy and balanced dish. For about seven years, Dash Diet has been chosen as the best diet that benefits our health. The magazine "Us news & world report" summarizes the rankings of the Mediterranean diet, which is only second.

There are parameters to evaluate the most reliable diet, such as nutritional characteristics, safety, effective weight loss, health benefits, and ease of execution.

You can reduce pressure by adopting a DASH diet (short for the diet to stop high blood pressure) and reducing sodium intake (especially in salt cooking and industry).

Both of these factors can reduce pressure, even if faced individually. However, the combination of diet and low sodium intake can provide the greatest benefit, contribute to the prevention of hypertension, and provide additional results related to regular physical activity practice.

The dash diet lowers pressure and focuses on meat, fish, legumes, and vegetables (eat before meals!), which helps you lose extra kilos. Find what you expect.

The effects of diet, prevent and normalize high blood pressure, and promote weight loss. Diets are based on food quality, not quantity and weight loss doesn't occur as quickly as other diets.

Do not make any major changes to your diet suddenly. Make small changes and don't abandon them. If these changes become a habit, incorporate a few more changes.

A plan that includes long-term and short-term goals and ideas for overcoming barriers, that is, factors that hinder dietary changes, will be more successful.

Dash Diet is a diet model designed to lower blood pressure and improve heart health. The Dash diet is also the right diet plan to lose healthy weight.

Start a DASH diet right now: it helps to prevent or control high blood pressure, but it's not just that. Because it has heart benefits, it can be used as a slim diet and is suitable for all nutritional needs.

CHAPTER ONE
ABOUT DASH DIET

This is the 9th record time DASH diet was among the best diets in the world according to the health report "US News".

From 2010, the DASH diet was selected annually as the number 1 among the most popular nutrition systems; in 2018 it won first place along with the Mediterranean diet, while for 2019 it is recommended immediately after it.

The "US News Health Report" ranking in the "Best Diet" category is created with the participation of over 20 experts, including dietitians, dietary consultants and doctors specializing in, among others in slimming and treating heart disease or diabetes.

As part of it, 41 diets were assessed for features such as protection against civilization diseases, ease of use, the effect on weight loss and the ability to maintain a lower weight. In terms of impact on health, the DASH diet scored 4.8 points out of 5!

The DASH diet is suitable for people of all ages, providing numerous beneficial effects and a drop in blood pressure after just 2 weeks!

DIET DASH - DIETARY APPROACHES TO STOP HYPERTENSION

The name of the DASH diet comes from the name of the study in which it was evaluated - it was titled "Dietary Approach to Stop Hypertension" - "Dietary Approaches to Stop Hypertension". They were carried out more than 20 years ago in support of the American National Institute of Heart, Lung and Blood-forming System (NHLBI), which is the body of the National Institute of Health (NIH).

Because untreated hypertension increases the risk of developing heart disease, heart attack, and stroke, the right nutritional strategy was to help reduce the risk of developing it. The diet has proved extremely effective and to this day there are more discoveries about its beneficial effects on health.

It has been proven, among others, that the DASH diet helps prevent the development of hypertension facilitates the improvement of an abnormal blood lipidogram, reduces the risk of developing cardiovascular diseases and type 2 diabetes, as well as general mortality, contributing to prolonged life.

The high effectiveness of the DASH diet is related to its design, reminiscent of the Mediterranean style diet on which it was modeled. However, the beneficial effect is mainly because sodium intake is reduced and potassium, magnesium, and calcium doses are increased.

It is possible thanks to limiting the consumption of industrial food, especially of animal origin and increasing the number of greens and other unprocessed plant products, especially cereals.

DASH DIET DEFINITION

DASH (Dietary Approaches to Stop Hypertension) has been designed by American researchers to reduce or prevent hypertension.

It is rich in fruits, vegetables, and whole grains, as well as low-fat or fat-free dairy products, fish, poultry, beans, seeds, and nuts. Fats and sugars are very limited.

DASH is a flexible meal plan that focuses on natural foods such as vegetables, fruits, whole grains, non-fat or low-fat dairy products, fish, chicken, beans, nuts, and vegetable oils (such as olive oil). All ingredients are effective in promoting health, including diet.

The DASH diet was not originally made to lose weight. But it is clear that factors that affect blood pressure (processed foods, trans fatty acids, excess sugar, etc.) also affect body weight. Studies have shown that people who continued DASH diets lost more weight in 8-24 weeks than other low-calorie diets.

The abbreviation of DASH is the acronym of Dietary Approaches to Stop Hypertension which means that it is a dietary program based on dietary results recommended by the expert group of a famous institution in 1997 to lower blood pressure.

The DASH healthy diet is a certified treatment for hypertension, heart disease, and kidney disease even without any medical help. Hypertension is also called the silent killer that has no previous symptom or warning.

The DASH diet completely emphasizes the correct nutrition of foods with the portion size and the right amount of nutritional value.

This diet plan is a combined plant-based diet that should be rich in whole grains, fruits, vegetables, nuts, seeds, meat, nuts, etc. It is also rich in dietary fiber, potassium, calcium, protein, and magnesium.

But it must be low in sodium, cholesterol, fatty dairy products. This perfect combination of diet is highly recommendable for the person who wants to prevent or control hypertension which also reduces the risk of contracting heart disease.

The functionality of these properly planned diets is classified into a logical category based on seven types of security: easy to follow, high nutritional value, short term weight loss results, effective and preventive management of diabetes, and various heart conditions.

MORE ON DASH DIET

The DASH project compared 3 different types of diet:

1 group followed normal eating habits; the second group saw an increase in the quantities of fruit and vegetables, while the third group had to follow the DASH dietary plan.

The results showed that both the second and the third groups were able to reduce blood pressure, but in the case of the DASH diet this result was achieved in just 2 weeks.

The second study, called DASH-Sodium, instead set itself the goal of verifying how lower sodium levels in the diet could affect blood pressure.

The study participants were divided into 2 macro-categories (one followed the DASH plan of the first project, the other the normal supply) and each macro-category was then divided into 3 further categories based on the sodium levels in the feed: over 3300 mg, about 2400 mg and 1500 mg of sodium.

The research results showed that a reduction in sodium levels showed a reduction in blood pressure for both macro-categories, and the greatest reduction occurred in the 1500mg-plane DASH combination.

DASH diet has been classified as the best and healthiest against hypertension and diabetes for 3 consecutive years.

It has been shown to reduce blood pressure and cholesterol, as it is also excellent to follow in the presence of some diseases, but it is ideal for keeping hypertension under control.

If your blood pressure rises above 120/80 even slightly, you may already notice some side effects.

The more blood pressure deviates from optimal values, the greater the risk to our health. Researchers began to investigate the causes of high blood pressure by analyzing single elements, such as calcium and magnesium, but none of those studies was able to arrive at certain results.

In America, there was then two key research supported by the NHLBI.

The first study, called DASH, analyzed the influence of each food on blood pressure and discovered that blood pressure was reduced following a diet low in saturated fats and cholesterol, and emphasizing instead the intake of low fruit, vegetables, and products of fat.

They then elaborated on a dietary plan, DASH precisely, which also included the intake of products based on durum wheat, poultry fish, and hazelnuts, while limiting red meat, sweets, and sugary drinks.

The plan was also rich in magnesium, potassium, and calcium, as well as protein and fiber.

DASH DIET STARTUP

The DASH diet was originally developed over twenty years ago at Harvard University in the United States and its main purpose was to control hypertension, a widespread disease in the adult population, and with serious consequences.

The DASH diet, thanks to the foods of which it is rich, presents a high quantity of vitamins, calcium, magnesium, potassium, fibers, and polyphenols.

It is a diet rich in fruits, vegetables, mostly whole grains, and low-fat dairy products. Dried fruits, legumes, seeds, fish, and white meat are also present in moderate quantities, while foods such as red meat, fried foods, and desserts are limited.

The first of the research concerning the DASH diet was carried out on 459 adults, with systolic pressure below 160 mmHg and diastolic blood pressure between 80 and 95 mmHg.

About 27% of the participants suffered from hypertension; about 50% were female and 60% were of African-American origin.

In the research three different diets were compared:

- The first included foods similar to those normally taken by the American population;
- The second was identical to the first, with the addition of fruit and vegetables;
- The third was the DASH diet.

All three diets included a daily sodium intake of 3,000 mg; none were vegetarians nor did they provide common foods in specific ethnic traditions.

The results were sensational. Those who followed both the diet with fruit and vegetable supplementation and the dash diet managed to lower the pressure, but it was the dash diet that achieved the best results, especially among people with hypertension.

Also, the pressure decreased almost immediately, within two weeks of starting the diet.

The second research concerning the dash diet focused on the effects of reduced-sodium consumption on blood pressure: the participants, divided into two groups, followed the dash diet and another diet that reflected normal Western diet, respectively.

In this second research 412 people were involved, to whom one of the two groups was randomly assigned, and who then had to stick to one of the three sodium levels expected for a month:

- The high level, that is the one consumed by the majority of Americans and equal to 3,300 mg per day,
- The average one, equal to 2,300 mg a day
- And the low one, equal to 1,500 mg a day.

The results showed that, by decreasing sodium consumption, the pressure subsided, regardless of the diet followed.

Furthermore, at each level, the pressure was lower in those who had followed the dash diet. The most significant decreases in blood pressure occurred among patients who followed the dash diet with a sodium intake of 1,500 milligrams per day.

Those who already suffered from hypertension previously experienced the sharpest decreases, but even those with prehypertension experienced significant decreases in blood pressure.

Jointly considered these two kinds of research show that it is important to decrease the consumption of sodium, regardless of the diet that is followed.

The winning combination, however, is represented by the dash diet and the decrease in salt and sodium consumption.

EFFECT OF DASH DIET

According to research conducted in 2017, the results of which are described in the Journal of American College of Cardiology, a low-sodium diet rich in heart-beneficial products, such as DASH, can lower too high blood pressure as well as commonly used drugs.

According to the Hypertension magazine, patients with elevated blood pressure following the DASH diet for 8 weeks resulted in a reduction in systolic pressure by an average of 6 mm Hg, and diastolic pressure by 3 mm Hg.

In hypertensive patients, the decreases in systolic and diastolic blood pressure were 11 and 6 mm Hg, respectively. The bodyweight of the subjects did not change.

The fact that the use of the DASH diet allows similar or even greater drops in blood pressure than when taking popular medications has been confirmed by the research discussed in the Journal of the American College of Cardiology.

They tested 2 versions of the diet - standard (2,300 mg sodium per day) and low-sodium (1,500 mg sodium per day). After 4 weeks, the reduction in blood pressure was higher compared to the high-sodium control diet, the higher the initial value of systolic pressure in patients:

above 150 mm Hg - 21 mm Hg less with low-sodium DASH, and 11 mm Hg less - with the standard; 140-149 mm Hg - 10 mm Hg less with low-sodium and standard DASH;

130-139 mm Hg -7 mm Hg less with low sodium DASH and 4 mm Hg less with standard, up to 130 mm Hg - 5 mm Hg less with low sodium DASH, 4 mm Hg less with the standard.

The DASH diet version richer in fat thanks to the use of full-fat dairy products proved to be as effective in reducing high blood pressure as the standard one - results from CHORI studies.

The results of which have been described in the American Journal of Clinical Nutrition, with the modified menu being slightly poorer in simple carbohydrates, incl. from fruit juices. After 3 weeks, it reduced the level of triglycerides and large and medium VLDL cholesterol molecules more effectively than the standard version of the diet.

The introduction of the DASH diet protects women against the development of heart disease, which was confirmed in studies from the "Archives of Internal Medicine".

Participants using menus that most met the diet requirements by 24% were less likely to get coronary heart disease and by 18% they had fewer strokes. Lower levels of C-reactive protein and interleukin-6 have been found in their blood, which are indicators of inflammation in the body.

The DASH diet reduces the risk of gout - a painful inflammatory disease of the joints (usually the big toe) caused by the accumulation of uric acid crystals in them (another place where they can accumulate are the kidneys - the effect is kidney stones).

Statistics show that almost 75 percent. patients with gout also have hypertension and more than 60 percent. metabolic syndrome is found.

In a survey lasting over 26 years conducted on over 44,000 men aged 40 and over, the rarer the occurrence of the disease was confirmed, the closer the daily diet was to the DASH recommendations.

Adhering to the recommendations of the DASH diet also reduces the incidence of depression in the elderly, which results from studies presented in 2018 at the annual congress of the American Academy of Neurology.

During the 6.5 years under study, it was shown that a diet closer to the ideal DASH recommendations reduces the risk of depression by up to 11 percent, and the more it resembles a Western-style menu, the more it promotes the development of this disease.

HABIT CHECKLIST OF DASH DIET

DASH diet is a new diet and a diet that you should follow throughout your life. If you don't follow it for several days, don't be discouraged and go back to the "right path" and continue to pursue your food goals.

Ask yourself why you are tempted. Was there a party? Did you feel stress due to work or family life? Find the cause of the temporary departure from the route and resume immediately after the dash diet.

Don't worry too much. Sooner or later, all those who follow the diet will seduce themselves, especially when they are still in the running-in phase. Remember that lifestyle changes are a process that can last a long time.

Ask yourself if you have done too much at once. In many cases, people trying to change their lifestyles are overkill. Try to change a few things at once. The change will be slower, but it is certainly the best way to do it.

Divide the process into many small steps. Doing so will not only invite you to do too much at once but also make it easier to change. A single difficult task can be broken up into smaller and simpler steps and created very easily.

Keep a diary. Use the agenda to keep track of what you eat and what you do. This makes it easier to understand where the problem is. Keep a diary for several days.

You may find yourself used to eat fatty foods while watching TV. In this case, you can start by keeping an alternative snack low in fat.

A diary can also help you determine if you have a balanced diet and have enough physical activity.

DOS AND CONS OF THE DASH DIET

Among the DOS we find:

- Lowering cholesterol and high blood pressure

- lose weight

- The organism is purified

- Prevent tumor

- Against the onset of diabetes

- Helps combat moisture retention

- It's a simple meal that doesn't require much time

- Vegetarians can also practice

- Also suitable for people suffering from celiac disease and lactose intolerance

IN THE CONS WE FIND:

- Give up sweets that are healthy but not easy for everyone

There are no special contraindications for the Dash diet. It is highly recommended not to eat without medical supervision

CHAPTER TWO
FEATURES OF DASH DIET

Dash diet feature is the complete removal of salt and a higher increase in the number of vegetables, proteins, and fruits.

The fat and sodium are reduced, cholesterol is reduced, hypertension is reduced, and weight loss and general health are improved.

Sugar and alcohol intake should also be reduced.

Have a healthy diet and a habit of sticking to the dash diet

TYPES OF DASH DIET

The DASH diet has 2 variants depending on its sodium content:

The standard DASH diet - max 2300 mg sodium per day

Low-sodium DASH diet - max. 1500 mg sodium per day

(1000 mg sodium is contained in 2500 mg table salt)

The first option is a diet that is poorer in sodium than the average consumption in developed countries (3500 mg or more).

While the second option, which lowers blood pressure most effectively, requires strict limitations even for products such as bread or cheese.

Processed food is the main source of sodium in the diet, which comes not only from table salt itself but also from food additives

DASH DIET LAWS

At the base of the Dash diet, there are some principles that we could summarize in: eating little of almost everything, without exceeding in any single element of the diet

Let's look at the cornerstones of these principles:

- Abolish the added sodium chloride (NaCl - kitchen salt)
- Abolish foods stored by sodium chloride (NaCl - table salt)
- Abolish alcohol consumption
- Encourage the consumption of foods rich in potassium, magnesium, and calcium
- Significantly reduce the consumption of foods rich in saturated/hydrogenated fats and cholesterol
- Favor the consumption of foods rich in essential fatty acids ω3
- Take protein in moderate amounts
- Reduce excessive glycemic loads (too many carbohydrates together)
- Reduce sweets and red meat, favor the consumption of white meat
- Make the right amount of milk to low-fat, skim milk, or yogurt
- Make the right amount of whole grains (pasta, rice, cereals, or bread)
- Abound in fish, vegetables (especially legumes), and fruit (especially nuts and fresh seasonal fruit)
- Use an oligo-mineral water

ADVANTAGES OF FOLLOWING THE DASH DIET

Dash diet has numerous advantages and it is considered the best diet ever. Here are the benefits of the dash diet

HELPS TO LOSE WEIGHT

The nutrients that this diet provides promote the proper functioning of the intestines and thus the digestive process.

It is also rich in dietary fiber, causing a feeling of fullness and extending the period between meals.

Finally, their exercise proposals follow the guidelines recommended by the American Heart Association to reduce overweight and combat sedentary lifestyles.

BETTER NUTRITION

DASH diets are all about a healthy diet, and most packaged foods contain excess salt and sugar.

FIGHTING HYPERTENSION

The main purpose of the dash diet is to provide nutrients such as magnesium, calcium, and potassium, reduce the presence of sodium, and lower blood pressure.

Various studies conducted to study its effects have been shown to be effective in patients with moderate to severe hypertension.

Their results are usually seen two weeks after adopting the diet.

CONTROL CHOLESTEROL

"Bad" cholesterol in the blood can combine with other substances and form plaques in the blood vessels.

These impede blood circulation and increase the risk of heart disease. Healthy fats, minerals and fiber in the dash diet increase the presence of "good" cholesterol and reduce the damage that causes the same name.

CANCER PREVENTION

Thanks to the high intake of vegetables and fruits and hence antioxidants, those who follow the Dash diet are at a lower risk of suffering from cancer.

LOWER RISK OF CARDIOVASCULAR DISEASE

Dash diet reduces the risk of stroke and cardiovascular disease and is associated with the high consumption of vegetables and fruits typical of this diet.

DASH is a balanced diet strategy that can be adopted to achieve a healthier diet and lifestyle.

DISADVANTAGES OF DASH DIET

DASH diet has some drawbacks. Losing weight using a diet plan without properly describing calories is not the best strategy.

First of all, it is important to create a caloric deficiency that is appropriate (not extreme, not too light) according to your metabolic needs. This does not mean that it is possible to adapt a low-calorie plan to the dash concept.

Others may find it difficult to adapt to all the fiber consumption recommended by the Dash Diet. To avoid swelling and physical discomfort, we recommend gradually adding foods rich in fiber, such as whole grains, fruits, and vegetables.

DASH DIET BELIEVERS

Especially for people who are suitable for the DASH diet. The dash diet was developed by the National Institutes of Health. It aims to help people suffering from high blood pressure lose weight by improving their diet.

Dash diet is mainly useful for people who want to lower their blood pressure because their blood pressure is too high. It is also recommended for people with cardiovascular disease or at risk. But it is useful for everyone, regardless of pressure level, to promote a healthy approach to nutrition.

In addition, the dash diet helps with weight loss and has many benefits for the human body. It lowers blood sugar and cholesterol and reduces the risk of stroke, high blood pressure, and heart disease.

IN SUMMARY

Due to confirmed health-promoting effects, it is recommended especially to people with problems such as:

- High blood pressure and high blood pressure

- Abnormal lipidogram - too high total and LDL cholesterol in the blood,
- Pre-diabetes and diabetes
- Overweight and obesity
- Metabolic syndrome
- Other risk factors for the development of cardiovascular diseases,
- Gout (arthritis),
- Kidney stones and kidney disease
- Constipation and digestive disorders.

IS DASH DIET FOR ALL

"The diet is richer than most Americans are accustomed to because it emphasizes eating more fruits and vegetables instead of processed foods.

Fiber is one of your best allies when it comes to losing kilos because fiber has the effect of getting bored.

Each year, the US magazine US News & World Report asks a team of medical professionals to rank about 40 diets. DASH has been selected as the best global diet for the eighth consecutive year, and there are good reasons for that.

Their rules are not crazy and food groups are not excluded. In general, it is a very healthy diet.

If you want to eat more fruits and vegetables (which we all should), DASH is a simple and healthy plan that almost everyone should follow.

More likely to consume more nutrients, which may also improve bowel movements

So the DASH diet is good for everyone.

CHAPTER THREE
THE SODIUM EFFECT

SODIUM PHRASES AND MEANING

Search for the following information about cans, boxes, bottles, bags, and other types of packaging.

- sodium

Sodium-free or salt / no salt less than 5 mg per serving

- Minimum sodium content up to 35 mg sodium per serving

- Low sodium up to 140 mg sodium per serving

- Up to 140 mg sodium per 100 g low sodium food

- Low sodium content Sodium at least 25% less than conventional versions

- The amount of sodium is half that of conventional sodium with less sodium

- If salt is not added during the preservation process, it will not be added (in fact, the food is completely free of salt)

- Less than 0.5 mg per serving without fat

- Lack of saturated fat Up to 1 g portion and up to 15% calories derived from saturated fat

- Less fat up to 3 ga part

- Low-fat at least 25% less fat than conventional versions

- Half the amount of fat compared to the traditional version

THE SODIUM PROBLEM

Table salt is one of the basic spices used for cooking and preserving food, and at the same time is the main source of sodium in our diet.

This component is necessary for the proper functioning of the body because it maintains optimal fluid volume and blood pressure affects the state of the cell and tissue hydration, is also responsible for the proper conductivity of nerve cells and the functioning of the muscular system.

Sodium deficiency in the body could therefore be dangerous to health, and in some situations, even to life.

Much more often, however, we have a problem with the consequences of excess sodium than its deficiency in the body.

Healthy people should consume no more than 1 teaspoon of salt from all sources per day (i.e. salt added to dishes and contained in ready-made products such as bread, sausages, cheese, salty snacks).

Meanwhile, studies carried out in Poland have shown that the average sodium consumption is 2-3 times higher than the demand, regardless of the age group of the respondents.

Prolonged consumption of excessive amounts of sodium can cause many serious diseases - including increases in blood pressure, which leads to heart attack and stroke, is also a direct cause of edema associated with water retention.

It can increase the loss of water in the urine, overloading the kidneys and the formation of kidney stones, as well as liver problems. Regularly exceeded sodium in the diet increases cholesterol, thereby increasing the risk of atherosclerosis

It is also associated with the development of diabetes, obesity, dementia, and osteoporosis. What's more, in recent years it has been explicitly confirmed that excessive consumption of salt and salt-preserved food are factors contributing to stomach cancer.

These types of diet errors can result in damage to the gastric mucosa,

To reduce the risk of developing diseases that are a consequence of excess salt, you should give up adding salt to your daily diet, limit the addition of salt during cooking and preparing food for consumption.

It is worth limiting the consumption of food containing large amounts of sodium - meats, canned meat and fish, rennet and blue cheese, silage, smoked products, marinated vegetables, soups and sauces, spice mixtures, broth cubes, salty snacks (chips, sticks, pretzels, crackers, nuts).

To be more aware of the salt/sodium content of individual foods, read labels carefully, and quantify your sodium content. If there is no such information, then the composition of the product will be helpful - the less salt in the product, the further place among the ingredients was placed.

When preparing homemade meals, the salt can be partially replaced with fresh or dried herbs (e.g. basil, oregano, thyme, rosemary, coriander, marjoram) and seasoning vegetables (peppers, garlic, parsley, dill, chives).

Instead of traditional salt, you can choose low-sodium (potassium or magnesium). In this way, we shape the habit of salty taste ourselves, while caring for our health.

SODIUM DEFICIENCY

Adult daily sodium demand is 1200-1500 mg. Today, sodium deficiency is very rare. The media is constantly running campaigns to reduce consumption of this element, including salt.

Salt is found in large quantities of food. However, the sodium concentration in the body may be too low. Usually, it is not a dietary problem but a health problem. The main causes of sodium deficiency are:

- Chronic diarrhea
- vomiting,
- Intense sweating
- Kidney problems
- heart failure
- Liver failure
- Adrenal dysfunction.

These are just a few of the situations that can lead to that shortage. Often, low sodium levels are observed in athletes after prolonged fatigue efforts. This situation occurs, for example, in a marathon runner.

In many cases, prolonged running at high temperatures can lead to prolonged sweating that can cause electrolyte disturbance. People who abuse laxatives are also at risk of sodium and other electrolytes falling.

If hyponatremia (low sodium concentration in the body) has already occurred, the following symptoms can be expected:

- Reduced concentration and memory,
- Loss of appetite
- Increased fatigue
- Headache,
- Lower blood pressure
- Sleepiness,
- Dizzy.

The above symptoms are associated with mild hyponatremia. Her heavy form has a more serious impact. A marked decrease in sodium (acute hyponatremia) can lead to brain edema, convulsions, and ultimately death.

EXCESS SODIUM IN THE BODY

Excess sodium in the body is called hypernatremia. Due to a poor diet, acute hypernatremia does not occur.

The cause may be excessive water loss from the body due to vomiting, diarrhea, or burns. Symptoms of acute hypernatremia are severe and include the following:

- Nausea,
- Muscle cramps
- Coma,
- Stroke.

The above conditions are very rare. Chronic hypernatremia is a more common problem, mainly due to a poor diet.

This condition is dangerous because it does not cause symptoms especially due to the body's ability to adapt. You can also develop later:

- High blood pressure,
- obesity,
- Nephrolithiasis
- Insulin resistance,
- Cardiac arrhythmia
- osteoporosis,
- Increased risk of stroke
- Increased risk of developing stomach cancer.

SODIUM-RICH PRODUCTS NOT RECOMMENDED ON A DASH DIET:

- Bouillon cubes and liquid spices,
- "Vegeta" type of spices
- Soy sauce,
- Miso paste,
- Olives,
- Capers,
- Dried tomatoes,
- Pickled cucumbers, pickled cabbage,
- Beet sourdough and other silages,
- Cheeses, especially feta, parmesan, rokpol,
- Sausages, especially dried ones,
- Salted and smoked fish,
- Cornflakes,
- Ready sauces,

- Fast food
- Powdered dishes,
- Salty snacks,
- Industrial sweets.

HOW TO REDUCE SODIUM

• If possible, select low sodium or non-sodium version foods and seasonings.

• Give preference to fresh or frozen vegetables, or vegetables that have been stored but have low sodium content or no added salt.

• Use white meat and fresh fish instead of seasoned, smoked, and preserved.

• Choose low sodium breakfast cereals.

• Do not overuse sausages (such as bacon or ham), salted foods (pickles, olives, sauerkraut), and special sauces (mustard, horseradish, ketchup, barbecue sauce).

• Cook rice, pasta, and cereal without salt. Do not use risotto, pasta, or cereal, which is usually very rich in salt.

• Choose foods that are low in sodium. It is famous for its frozen pizzas and dishes, processed or ready dishes, packeted or ready-made soups and salad dressings, and rich in sodium.

• Rinse canned tuna and beans to remove some of the sodium.

• Use spices instead of salt. Season your dishes with salt-free herbs, spices, lemons, limes, vinegar, or seasonal herbs on the kitchen and table. To get started, halve the amount of salt.

Reduce salt and sodium when eating out

• Ask how to prepare food. Ask to prepare without salt, sodium glutamate, or salt-containing ingredients. Most restaurants will meet your needs.

• Learn about words and expressions that indicate the presence of salt, such as "sottaceto", "stagionato", "smoked", "soy sauce", "broth".

• Move the salt shaker away.

• Moderate seasonings such as mustard, ketchup, pickles, and salty sauce.

• Choose fruits or vegetables instead of salty snacks.

• Compare labels

• Read food nutrition information and compare the amount of sodium in different products. Check the sodium content in milligrams and the RDA ratio (recommended daily allowance). I like foods that contain less than 5% of RDA sodium. Those containing more than 20% of RDA are considered high in sodium.

• Remember to check the amount of other important nutrients in the DASH diet. The label helps you choose foods that are low in sodium, saturated fat, transgenic fat, cholesterol, calories, and abundant potassium and calcium.

CHAPTER FOUR
DASH FOOD INTAKE

GOOD FOOD FOR DIET DASH

The Dash Diet does not exclude all types of food but is particularly recommended for seasonal fruits and vegetables, whole grains, low-fat dairy products, and main protein from white meat.

You can also eat fish (especially blue), legumes, oilseeds, and dried fruits. Extra virgin olive oil is recommended as a seasoning.

In summary, the following intakes are recommended on the Dash diet.

- Seasonal fruits and vegetables
- Whole grain
- lean dairy products
- White meat
- •Blue fish
- Legumes
- Oilseeds
- •Dried fruit
- Extra virgin olive oil

For water, it is recommended to drink one and a half liters or two.

Here are some things you can eat on a Dash diet:

- Prefer whole grains over grains and flour, not exceeding 3 meals a day.
- Vegetables and vegetables that are naturally rich in potassium and magnesium. 3 or more times a day.

- •fruit. Use as snacks and snacks if possible, and consume 2-3 servings per day when possible.
- Red meat, chicken, fish, always aiming for cuts and varieties of lean meat, always combined with vegetable side dishes. Favor fish that are rich in omega 3 as much as possible, keeping a total of two parts: 200g or less for meat and 300 or less for fish.
- Nuts, seeds, legumes are rich in essential fatty acids, magnesium, potassium, a total of 4-5 servings per week.
- I prefer milk and derivatives, obviously red and yogurt, but no more than two meals a day, preferably not daily.
- Fats and seasoning oils. Promote intake of extra virgin olive oil or oils rich in monounsaturated fatty acids up to 2-3 servings per day.
- Mainly displays fresh seasonal fruits and vegetables. Preference is given to tomatoes, carrots, broccoli, spinach, asparagus, pumpkins, fennel, apricots, oranges, tangerines, peaches, pineapples, plums, cherries, and strawberries. Because it is rich in potassium.
- Fine unrefined grains (whole bread and whole wheat pasta).
- Dairy products can be consumed as long as they are thin. Fat-free proteins such as legumes (lentils and beans), white meat, chicken breasts, and rabbits are preferred.
- Pole position bluefish.
- Low-fat yogurt is also good without adding exaggeration without adding sugar and nuts (oily seeds like almonds, walnuts, sunflower seeds).
- Drinking 1.5 liters of water a day is essential.

AVOIDABLE FOOD FOR DIET DASH

To be strongly limited or eliminated altogether:

- Desserts
- Fat food
- Red meat
- Salt
- refined sugars
- fried foods
- no caffeine
- no saturated fats

- Sausages and dried products
- Seasoned cheeses and fat cheeses
- Refined flour and baked or packaged products
- Trans fat, butter, cream, egg yolk, lard, and lard
- Pancetta
- Hot dog
- Cold cuts
- Canned soups
- Smoked foods and pickles

DASH DIET IN ACTION

The statistics speak for itself, just 30 days after the start of a new meal. Many people have already lost about 3.5 kg. Moisture retention and fat accumulation are reduced.

The most prestigious dietitians and dietician dentists now agree to blame the idea that weight loss is the result of iron fast.

In addition to the physical level (vitamin deficiency, development of metabolic disorders, nutritional deficiencies), the significant reduction in daily caloric intake imposed by some meals is also psychologically absolute. Because it turned out to be harmful

Because this type of meal based on deprivation is really difficult to withstand the famine bear for the reasons mentioned above, it is easy to quickly invalidate all the sacrifices and get back a few of them in a short time, A lost kilogram that is very difficult to follow.

For all these reasons, Dash Diet is suitable for both those who suffer from heart and circulatory problems and those who love a healthy diet and want to stay healthy without giving up.

TIPS TO START WITH DASH DIET

Undoubtedly, the first step to implementing the DASH diet is to eliminate salt and products with a high content from your daily menu. However, this does not mean giving up tasty meals.

You can try to learn how to cook by the recommendations of the DASH diet or use ready-made solutions, e.g. by ordering diet catering.

- Although the DASH diet is associated with many sacrifices, it does not have to be boring. It is very important that meals are not only rich in essential minerals, but also tasty and interesting.

People who have problems with the cardiovascular system or hypertension can eat herbal risotto with forest mushrooms, roasted pepper soup with roasted chickpeas, or a chocolate roll with blueberry cream.

The most important are the ingredients we will use to prepare the dishes and the way they are prepared

STRATEGIES FOR DEALING WITH THE DASH DIET

Fruit or vegetables a day must be a major food for you, add a portion for lunch and one for dinner. Rather than going immediately to whole grains, start with one or two days with this type of cereal.

The gradual increase in fruit, vegetables, and whole grains can also help prevent any swelling or diarrhea caused by those on a high fiber diet.

Reward successes and forgive mistakes. Reward yourself with a non-food treatment for your accomplishments: rent a movie, buy a book, or do something that satisfies you. Everybody gets upset, especially when they learn a new thing

Add a physical activity. Increase your physical activity with the start of the DASH diet. Combining healthy eating and physical activity makes blood pressure reduction more likely.

Get support if you need it. If you have problems following your diet, always report it to your doctor or dietician. You may have suggestions for dealing with the new diet in the best way.

SUCCESS TIPS ON DASH DIET

• The weight loss plan is based on proper diet and exercise (at least 2 and a half hours of mild to moderate cardiovascular activity).

The meal should be 60-70% of the meal plan, but exercise is the rest. Complying with both aspects is essential for a successful weight loss diet.

• Adjuvants can be added to meet the basic pillars of a weight loss diet plan.

Among these are psychotherapy, mindfulness, yoga exercises, natural satiety medicine (always prescribed by experts), electrotherapy, or electroacupuncture.

But always take into account that they are the main thing, food, exercise assistance

• Must have 5 or 6 set meals per day, no more than 3 hours between each intake (3 staples and 3 side meals).

• You need to drink 2 liters of liquid per day. Half of 60% of the liquid should be water and the rest should be an infusion, coffee, tea, natural lemonade, or defatted natural broth.

• All food groups must be eaten throughout the meal or meal plan, but some groups are small and frequent (sweets, alcohol, complex carbohydrates). Complex carbohydrates should be taken at breakfast or lunch if possible, not at dinner.

• Do not limit the amount of food, especially with non-fat vegetables and proteins. The menu should be changed as much as possible in the plan.

• The only light products that can be consumed in the loss period are low-fat dairy products, sweeteners sweetened (more natural is better), and whole grains (bread, rice, pasta). The rest are normal products.

• Cooking methods need to be changed. Do not always cook the same thing (grilled, baked, steamed, cooked, stewed with less olive oil, barbecue).

• In general, all kinds of seasonings, herbs, and spices can be used without salt abuse. None of the dishes give more calories to the dish, but give it more flavor.

• The menu needs to be enhanced. We should not deprive the pleasant appearance of food and the taste of diet food. You can eat very rich, delicious and very healthy.

• Insist on lifestyle changes and lead to anxiety rather than food. This is the success of getting goals and maintaining them over time.

• A regular check-up with your doctor is required (every 7 or 15 days). Placing more control makes it very difficult to maintain planning discipline and compliance.

It can be done by you, but it is much more difficult and the chances of success are greatly reduced.

• You must eat a satisfactory amount of food that is not full. If we are accustomed to eating a lot, we need to gradually reduce the portion we serve and fill more with fat-free protein (chicken, turkey, rabbit, fish, eggs, skim milk) and vegetables.

CHAPTER FIVE
ABOUT HYPERTENSION

High blood pressure is another way to call high blood pressure. It can cause serious complications and increase the risk of heart disease, stroke, and death.

Blood pressure is defined as the force that blood exerts on the vessel wall. This pressure depends on the work of the heart and the resistance of the blood vessels.

High blood pressure and heart disease are the biggest concerns in the world. The World Health Organization (WHO) suggests that growth in the processed food industry has increased the amount of salt that food carries around the world, which plays a very important role in hypertension.

Hypertension is a civilization disease and remains the most important risk factor for premature death worldwide. Blood pressure is associated with mortality and the incidence of cardiovascular disease (myocardial infarction, stroke, heart failure, peripheral arterial disease), and renal failure.

Data from the last 20 years indicate an increase in the prevalence of hypertension in Poland. According to the NATPOL 2011 study, the prevalence of hypertension among people aged 18-79 has increased over the past 10 years from 30 to 32 percent, or to about 9 million people. 1

HYPERTENSION - SYMPTOMS

However, whatever the cause, hypertension for many years usually has no symptoms. Sometimes, however, some symptoms may also appear in other diseases, which is why they are called non-specific for hypertension.

However, it can be assumed that the more symptoms you see in yourself, the more likely you are to have high blood pressure:

- Pressure in the head - occurs occasionally and usually has the character of a dull headache
- Dizziness
- Fatigue
- Epistaxis
- Sleep disturbance
- Nervousness
- Ailments of the heart - with hypertension, there is a distinct pounding of the heart, a feeling of pressure or tightness in its area
- Dyspnoea

It is worth checking if the pressure is normal, because when the symptoms begin to overlap, it may be too late to compensate for the losses that the body has suffered because of it.

EFFECT ON ARTERIAL HYPERTENSION

In these cases, the Dash diet is sufficient to control the increase in blood pressure.

It is less effective on secondary forms of hypertension (ie deriving from other disorders) or on those with a strong genetic predisposition. In these cases, it can be a valid aid to therapeutic strategy allowing to keep the pressure under control with fewer antihypertensive drugs.

Both in the preventive and therapeutic fields, the Dash diet to counter hypertension is essentially based on three fundamental points, such as reduction of sodium intake below 3-5 grams per day increase in potassium intake, with the consumption of fruits, vegetables, and whole foods control of body weight and limitation of alcohol consumption

It may seem difficult to limit the addition of salt to dishes. In reality, it is a habit.

The palate can be easily re-educated. With a gradual reduction of the contribution of kitchen salt to foods, it will get used easily. Finding quite pleasant dishes that until recently could have been tasteless.

Then the cooking salt can be substituted with products with low sodium content such as potassium chloride, aromas, or various spices, such as oregano, sage, rosemary, garlic, parsley, and chili.

It is also recommended to consume as much fresh produce as possible, avoid seasonings, sauces, and ready-made dishes.

DASH DIET FOR HIGH BLOOD PRESSURE

The pressure can be considered high even if it is only slightly higher than the minimum level of 120/80 mmHg.

The more the pressure increases, the more serious your health risks are.

The DASH diet is a food plan created by the American National Institute for Health. The goal of the DASH diet is the reduction of blood pressure through nutrition, without the use of drugs. Its full name is "Dietary Approaches to Stop Hypertension".

The DASH diet can also be used as a food plan for weight loss. The DASH diet proposes healthy eating and the reduction of salt consumption, or sodium in general.

WHAT IS PRESSURE OF THE BLOOD

Blood pressure is the pumping power in which the blood pushes the artery walls. Blood pressure is measured in units called millimeters of mercury.

There are two blood pressure values:

SYSTOLIC PRESSURE - is the blood pressure on the arteries when the heartbeats. In common parlance, it is also called high blood pressure.

DIASTOLIC PRESSURE - is the blood pressure on the arteries when the heart is relaxed between beats. In common parlance, it is called low pressure.

BLOOD PRESSURE VALUES

Blood pressure values are considered normal when the systolic pressure is less than 120 mmHg and the diastolic pressure is less than 80 mmHg. In popular language, therefore, when the high pressure is less than 12 and the low one less than 8.

- High blood pressure, hypertension, we have when the systolic pressure is equal to or greater than 140mmHg and the diastolic pressure equal to or greater than 90mmHg. In other words, high blood pressure above 14 and low blood pressure above 9.
- When the values are intermediate, i.e. the systolic pressure is between 120 mmHg and 140mmHg, and the diastolic pressure between 80mmHg and 90mmHg, the condition is defined as pre-hypertension.
- Even when blood pressure is slightly above normal it can be harmful to health.

American researchers, funded by the National Heart, Lung, and Blood Institute (NHLBI) have conducted two fundamental studies.

Their findings have shown that it is possible to decrease blood pressure by following a type of diet with very minimal saturated and total fat with low cholesterol, which gives greater importance to fruit, vegetables, milk, and low fat or fat-free derivatives.

This diet, the dash diet, also includes products based on whole grains, fish, white meat, and nuts. Compared to the normal diet diffused in the western world (but very similar to the Mediterranean model)

The quantities of lean red meat, sweets, sugar, and sweet drinks are reduced. Instead, it is rich in potassium, magnesium, and calcium, as well as protein and fiber.

The following table is an indication of the ideal composition of the dash diet.

Total fats	27% of calories
Saturated fats	6% of calories
Protein	18% of calories
Carbohydrates	55% of calories
Cholesterol	150 mg
Sodium	no more than 2,300 mg
Potassium	4,700 mg
Football	1,250 mg
Magnesium	500 mg
Fibers	30 g

The dash diet aims to keep the heart healthy by limiting saturated fat and cholesterol intake. At the same time, the consumption of nutrient-rich foods known for their hypotensive effect, especially minerals (such as potassium, calcium, and magnesium), proteins, and fibers increases.

DASH diet, which means: dietary treatment to curb hypertension, was created to cope with high blood pressure since it predisposes to a decrease in blood pressure levels systolic and diastolic without drugs.

HIGH BLOOD PRESSURE

Hypertension (HT) is defined as an increase in blood pressure on the walls of the arteries.

According to the Joint National Committee on Detection, Evaluation, and Treatment of High Blood Pressure, for good diagnosis of hypertension, it is necessary to confirm the abnormal values obtained in a first evaluation, by at least two subsequent determinations of blood pressure.

Blood pressure (BP) fluctuates between two values, the maximum, at the time of ventricular systole, and the minimum, at the time of diastole.

Normal values are found when systolic BP is less than 120mmHg and diastolic BP is 80mmHg.

Pre-hypertension is considered when the values are between 120 / 80mmHg and 140 / 90mmHg, and hypertension when these are equal to or greater than 140 / 90mmHg.

Normally the hypertension is asymptomatic, although in more advanced stages it can cause headaches, nausea or vomiting, confusion, and/or nasal bleeding. Also, untreated high blood pressure can lead to numerous diseases.

It is important to put a lot of emphasis on lifestyle changes, such as weight reduction in case of overweight or obesity, decrease in salt intake, increase in physical activity, stopping the consumption of toxic substances (alcohol and tobacco), and acquisition of adequate eating habits.

Since these can play a fundamental role in primary prevention and the treatment of high blood pressure. This is where the DASH diet can be of great help.

DISADVANTAGES OF HIGH BLOOD PRESSURE

Hypertension is the most common condition seen in primary care. As we have seen before, when it is not well controlled, HTA can lead to:

- Myocardial infarction
- Stroke
- Renal insufficiency
- Death

That is why early detection and an adequate approach are essential.

DASH DIET FOR BLOOD PRESSURE

The DASH diet is based on incorporating:

- **WHOLE GRAINS:** as the main source of energy and fiber, such as legumes and whole grains (bread, pasta, rice).
- **FRUITS AND VEGETABLES:** Because they are good sources of potassium, magnesium, and fiber.
- **SKIMMED MILK PRODUCTS:** Sources of calcium and protein. They have to be skimmed or low in fat because the consumption of saturated fat is reduced in the DASH diet.
- **LEAN MEAT, POULTRY, AND FISH:** Sources of protein and magnesium. The consumption of red and processed meats will be avoided.
- **OILS:** Olive oil and margarine.

Therefore, the DASH diet is characterized by its high content of fruits, vegetables, and dairy products and the inclusion of whole grains, fish, and low amounts of sweets and sugary drinks.

It stands out for limiting the consumption of sodium, saturated fats, Trans fats, and cholesterol, promoting the consumption of fiber, potassium, magnesium, and calcium.

It is believed that it is the whole food model, rather than a specific food or nutrient that produces this reduction in blood pressure.

As the name implies, this diet was designed to lower high blood pressure, even so, other benefits were subsequently observed, such as lowering levels of LDL cholesterol or bad cholesterol.

With which, we could affirm that the dash diet is ideal to prevent cardiovascular diseases since it reduces these two risk factors.

IMPACT OF THE DASH DIET ACCORDING TO BASELINE BLOOD PRESSURE

Reduction of sodium levels and the DASH diet (Food approaches to stop high blood pressure), a diet rich in fruits, vegetables, low-fat dairy products, low cholesterol and saturated fatty acids, lowers blood pressure.

They know the results of these dietary interventions according to baseline blood pressure levels.

In this study, three comparisons are made based on diet and sodium levels. First, high sodium levels are compared with low sodium levels, then the DASH diet versus the control diet (low fruit and vegetable diet and with the amount of cholesterol and average fatty acids consumed in the US) and finally the two interventions.

The DASH diet and low sodium levels versus control diet and high sodium levels. The primary objective is the reduction of systolic blood pressure, and the secondary objective is the reduction of diastolic blood pressure, based on stratified patients according to their baseline blood pressure.

This is a secondary analysis of the DASH-sodium study, where adults with prehypertension and stage 1 hypertension, without antihypertensive treatment, were randomized to receive a DASH diet or control diet and different levels of sodium consumption.

First, the participants underwent a 2-week test phase where they fed the control diet and high sodium levels, then were randomized to the control diet or the DASH diet.

In the diet to which they were assigned they consumed low, medium or high levels of sodium (50, 100 or 150 mmol/day) at an increasing dose for 4 weeks each dose with a 5-day wash period where they were fed with the diet.

They are normally consumed. The order of consumption of sodium levels was randomized following a cross model.

The baseline strata of systolic blood pressure (SBP) were <130, 130 to 139, 140 to 149, and ≥ 150 mmHg and diastolic blood pressure (PAD) were <80, 80 to 84, 85 to 89, and ≥ 90 mmHg.

Of the 412 participants, 57% were women, and 57% were black, the average age was 48 years, and the mean blood pressure was 135/86 mmHg.

In the context of the control diet, sodium reduction (from high to low) was associated with an average SBP difference of -3.20, -8.56, -8.99, and -7.04 mmHg across the respective PAS strata listed previously.

In the DASH diet, sodium reduction (from high to low) was associated with a decrease in SBP of -0.88 mm Hg, -3.29 mmHg, -4.90 mmHg, and -10.41 mmHg.

In the high sodium group, the DASH diet versus the control diet was associated with a blood pressure difference of -4.5, -4.3, -4.7, and -10.6 mmHg.

The combined effects of the low-sodium DASH diet versus the high-sodium control diet were -5.3, -7.5, -9.7, and -20.8 mmHg.

The authors conclude that the combination of reducing sodium levels and the DASH diet lowered SBP across the entire range of pre and stage 1 hypertension, with progressively greater reductions in higher levels of baseline SBP.

The reduction of SBP in adults with high levels of SBP ($\geq$ 150 mmHg) was surprising and reinforces the importance of reducing sodium levels and the DASH diet in these high-risk groups

RULES TO FOLLOW

Although developed to lower blood pressure, this diet plan brings several benefits to the body.

Dash diet is recommended for weight loss because it is low in calories and rich in water and fiber, while it is low in monosaccharides and saturated fats.

The rules for the dash diet are as follows:

• Reduce salt to a minimum. Healthy subjects should not exceed 2300 mg. For subjects suffering from high blood pressure, the dose is 1500 mg. Like aromas or spices, reduce consumption of sausages, ripened cheese, and packaged products.

• Get plenty of fresh, seasonal fruits and vegetables, whole grains, and legumes, and are naturally low in sodium.

• Try dried fruits, oilseeds, extra virgin olive oil and blue fish rich in polyunsaturated fatty acids that have beneficial effects on the cardiovascular system.

• prefer foods rich in magnesium and potassium that regulate blood pressure

• Avoid foods rich in mono-saccharides, saturated fats, high sodium, salted or salted water, and smoked foods such as red meat, sausages and desserts.

• Avoid seasonings and sauces such as cream, mayonnaise and soy sauce.

• Drink 1.5 to 2 liters of water a day and prefer something with less sodium.

DASH AND WEIGHT LOSS

The original DASH diet was not originally designed for weight loss and was relatively rich in refined grains and starchy foods.

Since weight loss in a healthy and balanced way is important for many people, it was necessary to create a clear weight loss plan based on fruits and vegetables, low-fat and non-fat dairy products, nuts and beans And seeds.

As such, the diet has been modified, including balanced diets and snacks rich in real food (fruits and vegetables), and "good" fat-rich foods that are rich in protein and relieve a healthy heart and hunger.

The important caveat that I want to emphasize is the balanced amount of protein that maintains muscle mass at an optimal level, thereby avoiding metabolic slowdown.

The vegetable foods included in this diet are the principle of antioxidants and a powerful source of healthy heart fat, which can reduce oxidation and inflammation.

A diet rich in vegetables and fruits supports a healthy intestinal flora that makes our bodies healthy.

Therefore, the DASH diet plan offers a complete lifestyle program that improves heart health by lowering blood pressure and cholesterol while at the same time promoting weight loss.

HOW TO LOSE WEIGHT WITH THE DASH DIET

If you have to lose weight keep in mind that it is enough to lose a few pounds to see the risk of suffering from hypertension and other serious health problems diminish. In other words: it is better not to put on weight.

Recent research has shown that it is possible to lose weight if you follow the dash diet and reduce sodium consumption.

In research conducted on 810 people, a third of them learned to reduce sodium consumption and to follow the DASH diet daily, at the minimum calorie level, without forgetting healthy physical activity.

Within 18 months, the participants lost weight and were able to control the pressure more easily.

We remind you that the dash diet probably includes more portions of foods based on fruits, vegetables and whole grains than the diet you are used to.

This diet is high in fiber, so in some people, it can cause bloating and diarrhea. To avoid these problems the intake of fruits, vegetables and whole grains should be gradually increased.

Instead, the secret to reducing the amount of salt in the diet is to eat intelligently.

Only a small amount of the salt we take is represented by cooking salt, the salt contained in the salt shaker, so to speak, and only very small amounts of sodium are present in the non-preserved foods.

It follows that the main source of sodium is processed and preserved foods, so it is important to read the labels carefully and choose products with low sodium content. The list of sodium-rich foods is surprisingly long, including:

- The leavened products and the yeast itself,
- Some cereals,
- Seasoned foods,
- Monosodium glutamate and some antacids.

The dash diet was not expressly designed to lose weight, but it also lends itself effectively to this need; we also remember that losing even a part of one's overweight allows concrete benefits from the health point of view.

It is rich in low-calorie foods, such as fruit and vegetables. You can further decrease your caloric intake by replacing high-calorie foods, such as sweets, with more fruit and vegetables: by doing so it will be easier to achieve the goals of the dash diet.

If you are trying to lose weight, try to reach a lower caloric threshold than you normally consume: the best way to lose weight is:

- Lose weight gradually
- Do more physical activity
- And follow a balanced diet, low in calories and fat.

Don't forget to follow these tips to save other calories:

- Use non-fat or low-fat condiments, so the butter must be removed.
- Halve the quantity of seed oil, margarine, mayonnaise or sauces, or, if they exist, choose the lean versions.
- Gradually get used to smaller portions.
- Choose skimmed or partially skimmed milk or derivatives.
- Check the labels, to compare the amounts of fat contained in packaged foods: foods that claim to be lean or fat-free can sometimes have higher calorie content than normal ones.
- Moderate amounts of very sweet foods, such as cakes, processed yoghurts, candies, ice creams, puddings, and carbonated drinks and fruit juices.

- When you eat yogurt (lean), add some fruit.
- To make a snack, choose a fruit, a few cut and clean vegetables, unsalted and not too greasy popcorn or rice cakes.
- Drink water or tonic water, flavored with a slice of lemon or lime.

WHAT TO DO IF YOU CAN'T LOSE WEIGHT

If it's difficult to lose weight with a healthy diet like Dash, you'll need to develop some strategies.

• Small parts

• Increase in fiber consumption

• Exercise for at least 30 minutes a day to maintain weight, or 60 minutes if weight is needed.

DASH DIET AND PHYSICAL EXERCISE

By combining the DASH diet with regular physical activity programs such as running and swimming, you can lose weight and maintain long-term results. 30 minutes a day of moderate intensity physical activity can become a true panacea.

If it is slightly higher than your average pressure, you may just walk at an active pace for about 30 minutes every day, without having to rely on medication.

If you take medicine for high blood pressure, moderate physical activity 30 minutes a day increases the effect of the medicine and makes you feel better.

Even if you do not suffer from high blood pressure, physical activity can help you stay healthy.

If you tend to sit while you have normal blood pressure, you are more likely to suffer from high blood pressure, especially with aging, overweight, obesity, and diabetes.

To start a physical activity program, simply walk around the block for 15 minutes once in the morning and evening.

Build your program little by little and set new goals so you don't lose your motivation. Keep in mind that trying to do everything right away will force you to stop because it can cause health problems.

If you are suffering from chronic health problems, or if your family has a history of heart disease at a young age, it is recommended that you seek advice from your doctor before starting an exercise program.

Make a plan and respect it

Ask your friends and family if you want to get along with them. Mutual motivation helps you avoid giving up.

Do not fossilize in a single activity. Try different activities to keep your daily efforts from focusing on parts of your body.

Give my goals

Give yourself ward beauty. At the end of each month's exercise, reward yourself with gifts, dresses, records, new books, and things that will help you stay trusted in the program. But don't reward yourself for food.

DASH DIET EXERCISES

It is obvious by researches and represented by the fact that weight control increases the cardiovascular benefit obtained by following the DASH diet, emphasizing that this indicates how important it is that weight loss and exercise is included in any program that includes a change in the lifestyle of people who has higher blood pressure

TYPES OF DASH DIET EXERCISE

TO WALK

Needless to say, one of the most effective exercises to burn calories and therefore lose weight is the banal walk.

If you have to go downtown or do the shopping, consider going there on foot if you can, you will thank your partner and your heart.

BIKING

And if the supermarket or workplace is not very close, the bike is an efficient means of economic transport, and that will make you feel good and healthy.

TAKING THE STAIRS

Instead of taking the lift, we do all the times we can the stairs, the environment and our hearts will be in thanks.

JUMPING JACK

Jumping jack is an exercise often used in the army also known as New Zealand push-ups.

It is often used as a free-body aerobic exercise during warm-up. Extend your legs and arms, and then jump over, gathering your knees towards your chest and pushing your arms down.

FRONT DIVE

Imagine we have a thread that starts from the top of the head that pulls upwards.

Slowly round the spine, vertebra after vertebra, trying to go forward and touch the floor with your hands.

With this movement, we stretch the column well.

SPINE TWIST

Sitting well on the ground, arms outstretched to the outside.

We rotate the chest, neck and head.

Imagine screwing the spine in one movement towards the other.

LATERAL RAISE

This exercise is particularly useful for toning the shoulders.

Grab light dumbbells (or two half-full bottles of water, or two 1/2-liter bottles, off to the imagination) start with your hands at your sides, keep your elbows slightly bent, and raise your arms sideways at shoulder level.

The movement must be fluid and soft, you must not feel any pain. You must perform it smoothly. Repeat 5-7 times, but don't overdo your body. The watchword is being gradual

CROSSOVER CRUISE

This exercise works on the diagonal abdomen.

Walk your back with your knees bent and your feet on the floor.

Next, place your right ankle on your left knee and place your hands behind your head.

Open the elbow, rotate the trunk slowly, lift the inhalation when returning to the ground, and bring the left elbow towards the exhaled right knee.

Alternate the sides.

PLANKING

This is one of the best exercises to keep your abdomen in order and stable.

Some strength is required, but it can be done calmly.

We lie down on the floor leaning on the forearms.

At this stage, we are resting and our feet are lying on the ground.

Next, put the lever on the floor with the lower limbs and raise the pelvis so that the back is completely straight.

Repeat at least 5 times by contracting the abdominal muscles and maintaining the position for 30-60 seconds.

HALF ROLL DOWN

Seated on the ground, the column is rotated halfway.

To perform the movement well, it is necessary to pull the navel back, slowly start to rotate the pelvis until you get to the maximum flexion of the lumbar spine, keeping shoulders and head erect.

SIDE BEND

Feet firmly planted in the ground, active abs and shoulders far from the ears.

Make a tilt movement first to the left then to the right

SIDE BEND ABDOMINAL VACUUM

It is an exercise derived from yoga and that strengthens the belly muscles, thus avoiding prolapse.

Standing position, hands on the hips and slightly bent legs. Take a deep breath and breathe out by tilting your torso forward, letting all the air out of your lungs and pulling your belly back.

In this position we hold the breath for 5 - 6 seconds, breathe in and start again, repeating a dozen times. It can also be done on all fours, a typical American version.

CHAPTER SIX
DASH DIET PROCESS

DASH DIET SHOPPING

Compliance with the DASH diet begins with the food you purchase. Before shopping:

Make a list. Decide what you will prepare next week and write down the necessary ingredients.

First, eat. Do not buy food when you are hungry. If you buy when you are hungry, everything looks attractive, making it difficult to resist fat and sodium-rich products.

Don't forget to plan breakfast and snacks. If you have a list at hand, you are less likely to be tempted by unhealthy food.

PAY ATTENTION TO THE DASH DIET WHEN SHOPPING

While at the grocery store, the large display and offer price can get your attention. Follow these tips to concentrate on the food recommended on the DASH diet.

BUY FRESH FOOD

Fresh food is a healthier option because it contains less sodium and less sugar and fat. Fresh foods tend to contain more vitamins, minerals and fiber than the packaged version.

BUY ON BOTH SIDES

There are many products suitable for the DASH diet in the central passage, but most of the time must be spent in the outer passage.

In the outer passage, you will find fresh ingredients, low-fat dairy products.

PLEASE READ THE LABEL

Most packaged foods in the United States have labels with nutrition information to help you determine how they fit into your diet. Daily intake of low-sodium foods is less than 5% per meal.

Look for low sodium and low-fat products. Compare similar items and select ones that are low in sodium, fat, and calories.

INCREASE DASH FOOD INVENTORY (DIET THERAPY TO STOP HIGH BLOOD PRESSURE).

If you have healthy food at hand, you are more likely to prepare a healthy dish. Try putting these items in the kitchen:

FRUITS

Choose from a variety of fresh fruits such as apples, oranges and bananas. Add variety with apricots, dates and berries. Choose canned fruits with their own juices, not syrup, and frozen fruits without added sugar.

VEGETABLES

Purchase fresh vegetables such as tomatoes, carrots, broccoli, and spinach, frozen vegetables, and canned foods. Choose frozen vegetables without salt, butter, or sauce. Choose low sodium canned vegetables.

LOW FAT DAIRY PRODUCTS

When buying milk, buttermilk, cheese, yogurt and sour cream, look for low-fat dairy products.

DASH DIET

BACK EXTENSION

With this exercise, you can tone and firm the buttock muscles.

Lie with your stomach on the floor face down.

Push with your lower back to lift your chest a few inches from the floor.

Your hands will be resting on your head.

Return to position, wait about twenty seconds and repeat the exercise.

KICKBACKS

This exercise is particularly indicated for the toning of the triceps which is that muscle located posteriorly in the arm (antagonist of the biceps).

Bend forward with your back straight and your abs well-stretched (like the greeting of judo to understand)

Start with light weights and bent elbows pointing your hands backward to engage the triceps to straighten your elbows. Excellent as dash diet exercises.

GRAIN

Buy whole-wheat bread, bagels, pita, cereals, rice, pasta, crackers, tortillas. Compare labels and select products with low sodium content.

NUTS, SEEDS, LEGUMES

Almonds, nuts, beans, lentils, chickpeas and sunflower seeds are some of the healthy options. But get varieties with no salt or low salt content.

RED MEAT, CHICKEN AND FISH

Choose a choice of lean meats such as skinless fish, chicken, turkey, pork loin, extra light ground beef, ground beef or sirloin. Look for poultry that has not been injected with fat or broth. Choose canned fish and meat with low sodium. Limit processed or processed meat such as cold meat.

SEASONINGS AND SPREADS

Herbs, spices, flavored vinegar, sauces, and olive oil can add flavor to your diet without excessive salt. Select the low or reduced sodium version of the seasoning.

USE APPROPRIATE KITCHENWARE

With kitchenware and appliances, you can easily track your DASH diet. Useful articles include the following:

NON-STICK KITCHENWARE

Non-stick cookware reduces the need to use oil or butter when baking meat or vegetables.

The vegetable vaporizer that fits in the bottom of the vegetable vaporizer pan makes it easy to cook vegetables with low nutrient loss and no added fat or calories.

Spice grinder or garlic press. These items promote the addition of flavor to the food and reduce reliance on salt.

USE HEALTHY COOKING TECHNIQUES

Unhealthy cooking habits can interfere with other efforts to follow the DASH diet. Use the following tips to reduce sodium and fat.

Choose a little taste. Use herbs, spices, flavored vinegar, onions, chili, raw ginger, lemon, garlic or garlic powder, or soup that does not contain sodium to improve the taste without adding salt or fat.

RINSE THE FOOD

Rinse canned beans and vegetables before use to remove excess salt.

PAY ATTENTION TO THE SOUP

Cook mushrooms, onions or other vegetables in a low sodium bouillon in a non-stick frying pan. But even a low sodium bouillon can contain a lot of sodium, so a healthy oil like olive oil may be a better option.

REPLACE WITH LESS FAT

Replace dairy products with low-fat or non-fat versions of whole milk.

REDUCE MEAT CONSUMPTION

Prepare casserole and casserole with just two-thirds of the meat required in the recipe, and add vegetables, brown rice, tofu, bulgur or whole wheat pasta.

If you normally cook or bake in a way that requires a lot of fat and salt, don't be afraid to change the recipe. Try spices and alternatives. Try diversifying the recipes that you can't usually do. You can happily be surprised

STARTING A DASH DIET

Getting started is very simple: for the dash diet, there is no need for special foods or even particularly elaborate recipes. You can start by checking if the dash diet resembles your current eating habits.

For a day or two make a list of everything you eat and check whether or not it follows our advice: in this way you will be able to understand what changes you need to make in choosing foods.

Remember that on some days the foods you take can increase the portions of a specific food group, and then decrease those of another group.

Similarly, on some days you may take too much sodium, but don't worry. On average, do not deviate too much from the dash diet instructions and the recommended sodium threshold.

The whole family can follow the dash diet instructions without any problems, based on their calorie needs when preparing different parts.

The dash diets, in combination with other lifestyle changes, help not only prevent high blood pressure but also manage blood pressure.

In this regard, the following is recommended:

• reach the proper weight, maintain it,

• Perform your favorite physical activity regularly,

• If you are not abstinent, consume alcohol moderately (1 cup for women and 2 for men).

WORKABILITY OF DASH DIET

The basis of this slimming diet is the elimination of salt, instead of increasing the consumption of fruit, vegetables and proteins.

In other words, less fat, less sodium, less swelling, less hypertension and less cholesterol with weight loss and improved overall health.

The DASH diet is constituted by two moments: the first phase lasts 14 days and aims to eliminate carbohydrates and fats replacing them with proteins, then follow a consolidation phase in which starchy vegetables must be reduced to keep the weight reached and to lower blood sugar and cholesterol levels.

So, the basis of this diet is not so much the calculation of calories but a greater consideration of what kind of food you choose to lose weight.

COOKING FOR DASH DIET

A little attention in the kitchen can further improve the quality of your meal.

With a good non-stick frying pan, you can use less or no oil/butter when cooking.

With a steamer, you can store all the valuable substances in vegetables and cook them quickly without seasoning.

Instead of frying, cook, roast or fry on the grill. Use moderate amounts of smoked or salted meat to remove excess fat from veal, pork and white meat.

Cook fish in foil to avoid dispersing aromas and juices.

Blow onions, mushrooms and other vegetables with a small amount of salty soup or water instead of butter or oil.

Instead of fat-rich ones, use skim milk derivatives such as fresh skim cheese or low-fat sour cream.

To taste the dish without adding salt or fat, onion, herbs, spices, flavored vinegar, fresh pepper, fresh or powdered garlic, raw ginger, lemon, lime, a little salty soup, or Use a small amount of low sodium soy sauce.

Add herbs, spices, or lemon juice to the vegetables.

Rinse canned foods such as tuna, legumes or vegetables before use to remove some of the excess salt.

Half the amount of sugar in the dessert to be prepared, and season it with a little cinnamon, nutmeg, vanilla, fruit and sweeten.

Prepare roasted or casserole using only two-thirds of the meat listed in the recipe. The remaining third can be replaced with vegetables, rice, tofu, bulgur or pasta.

If you like to make traditional and ethnic dishes that require a lot of fat and salt in the kitchen, don't be afraid to change the recipe.

Be creative: use spices, change ingredients and try new recipes. You may feel happy about your work.

HANDLING BARRIERS AND SLIDES IN DASH DIET

Take your time and think about the factors that hinder your path to success. These are called barriers. And if you think about these barriers now, you can plan what to do if they appear.

An example of a barrier is eating at a restaurant. If you do this frequently, it is wise to plan how you will follow the dash plan while dining out. Possible solutions are:

Reduce the frequency of eating out.

Look at the menu in advance, find what you can eat, and follow the meal plan.

Find a new restaurant that offers vegetarian and low-fat dishes.

It is quite normal to try something and quit yourself after interrupting it. Many people need to try many times before achieving their goals.

If you want to give, don't waste energy that makes you feel bad about yourself. Remember why you want to change, think about the progress you made, plant your encouragement, and talk to yourself to slap your back. Then you may want to try again.

Most people seek help when faced with barriers. Talk to your family and friends to see if someone wants or encourages you to eat healthy food with you.

Don't forget a small reward. If you have something to aim for, you can get on the right track.

How to get support

With a lot of support, it's easy to change your diet. For example, if your family says you like getting healthier, you might want to keep going the right way. Other ways to get support are:

Collaborate with partners. I am motivated to know that someone shares the same goal.

Your friends and family can eat healthy food with you. They can encourage you by telling you how you praise for making a big difference.

Join a class or support group. People in these groups often have some of the same barriers as you.

Don't forget to reward yourself. When you reach the goal, reward yourself. Purchase a new healthy cookbook.

Go to the cinema. Or take a moment. Do everything you need to remember that you are achieving your goals. Succeeded!

Full fill

Starting a new project can be frustrating, such as having a healthy diet and then having to interrupt to get sick, travel, bored, etc. His goal is to resume habits and make it part of everyday life.

Remember that you can't make a habit from one day to the next. Even if there is a slip on the road, keep to that custom. Every day is going in the right direction, as it can take up to 3 months to build habits.

Do not hate yourself or feel guilty when you have a slip. Think of it as a learning experience. Determine what happened. Why did it stop? Think about how to get on track. Learn from your slip so that you can continue towards a healthy eating goal.

CHAPTER SEVEN
DASH - MENU AND ITS COMPOSITION

In the DASH diet, it is important to control the portion size, limit the intake of sodium, animal fats, added fat and sugar. The menu is varied and balanced. It provides increased amounts of potassium, calcium and magnesium, as well as fiber, as well as the standard proportions of energy ingredients recommended in a balanced diet.

CHARACTERISTICS OF THE STANDARD DASH

- energy diet : 2100 kcal
- Protein: 18 percent
- Fat energy : 27% Energy Saturated
- Fat : 6% energy
- Carbohydrates: 66% Energy
- Fiber: 30 g
- Cholesterol: 150 mg
- Sodium: 2,300 mg
- Potassium: 4,700 mg
- Calcium: 1,250 mg
- Magnesium: 500 mg.
- Mortar instead of the salt shaker

On the DASH diet, it is the best solution that will make one of the healthiest ways of nutrition even more beneficial.

DASH DIET - A MENU OF 2,100 KCAL

The daily DASH diet plan with a standard calorie and sodium content is presented in a simple form of the recommended number of servings of products from individual food groups:

Cereal products: 6-8 servings,

Vegetables: 4-5 servings,

Fruit: 4-5 servings,

Lean dairy products: 2-3 servings,

Lean meat, fish, eggs: max. 6 servings,

Nuts, stones, legumes: 4-5 servings per week,

Oils and fats: 2-3 servings,

Sweets and sugars added: max. 5 servings per week

1 PORTION corresponds to:

Cereal products: 1 slice of bread; 30 g dry flakes; 1/2 cup cooked rice, cereal, or pasta;

Vegetables: a cup raw vegetables; then 1/2 cup vegetables in pieces or ground; 1/2 cup of vegetable juice 100 percent;

Fruit: 1 medium fruit; 1/2 cup small or ground fruit; 1/4 cup dried fruit; 1/2 cup fruit juice 100%

Lean dairy products: 1 cup milk or fermented milk drinks; 40 g yellow cheese;

Lean meat, fish, eggs: 30 g cooked meat or fish; 1 egg;

Nuts, stones, legumes: 1/3 cup or 40 g nuts; 2 tablespoons of peanut butter; 2 tablespoons or 20 g seeds and oilseeds; 1/2 cup cooked legume seeds;

Oils and fats: 1 teaspoon oil or soft margarine; 1 tablespoon of mayonnaise; 2 tablespoons salad dressing;

Sweets and sugars added: 1 tablespoon of sugar, jam or honey; 1/2 cup milk ice cream; 1 cup lemonade or other sweetened drinks.

How to prepare fish on the DASH diet? Salt the skin only, and replace most of the salt with lemon juice, herbs and hot peppers.

DASH DIET - MENU 1600, 2600 AND 3100 KCAL

The DASH diet menu is easily adapted to individual caloric needs, e.g. for men or sports. Additional doses of energy and necessary nutrients will be filled with a correspondingly increased daily number of servings of individual food products DASH DIET PLAN - 1600 KCAL PER DAY

Cereal products: 6 servings,

Vegetables: 3-4 servings,

Fruit: 4 servings,

Lean dairy products: 2-3 servings,

Lean meat, fish, eggs: 3-6 servings,

Nuts, stones, legumes: 3 servings per week,

Oils and fats: 2 servings,

Sweets and sugars added: 0 servings.

The DASH diet is a menu based on low sodium products. Instead of cured and store meats, it's best to choose those baked, fresh, homemade, prepared with lean meats.

DASH DIET PLAN - 2600 KCAL PER DAY

Cereal products: 10-11 servings,

Vegetables: 5-6 servings,

Fruit: 5-6 servings,

Lean dairy products: 3 servings,

Lean meat, fish, eggs: 6 servings,

Nuts, stones, legumes: 1 serving,

Oils and fats: 3 servings,

Sweets and sugars added: max. 2 portions

On the DASH diet, the addition of salt to meat dishes is best replaced by a rich mixture of pepper, spices and herbs.

Thanks to them, food will not only be aromatic and tasty but also healthier and easier to digest.

DASH DIET PLAN - 3100 KCAL PER DAY

Cereal products: 12-13 servings,

Vegetables: 6 servings,

Fruit: 6 servings,

Lean dairy products: 3-4 servings,

Lean meat, fish, eggs: 6-9 servings,

Nuts, stones, legumes: 1 serving,

Oils and fats: 4 servings,

Sweets and sugars added: max. 2 portions

30 DAYS DASH MEAL PLAN

DAY 1

BREAKFAST: EGG TOAST WITH SALSA
SERVINGS: 2

INGREDIENTS

- 1 large raspberry tomato
- 1 tablespoon of finely chopped onion
- chili to taste
- 2 teaspoons of lime juice
- 2 slices of bread (e.g. toasted bread, brioches, challah or bread)
- 2 teaspoons of butter and 1 teaspoon of oil
- 2 eggs
- fresh basil or coriander

PREPARATION

Heat the oven to 180 degrees C. Burn the tomato, peel and cut into cubes. Add finely chopped onion and chili pepper, season with a pinch of salt-free seasoning mixes and drizzle with lime juice.

Carve out the pulp from the center of the bread and fry the slices until golden brown in a pan in butter and olive oil.

Turnover, insert eggs into the centers, season with salt-free seasoning mixes. Next, put the tomatoes and put in the oven (if the panhandle is not heat-resistant, you can wrap it in aluminum foil).

Bake for about 10 minutes until the egg whites are cut. Serve with fresh basil or coriander.

LUNCH: SMOKED SALMON PITA BREAD, EGG CREAM AND GORGONZOLA CHEESE WITH PISTACHIO TOPPING

SERVINGS: 2 People

INGREDIENTS

- 150 gr of smoked salmon
- 100 ml of liquid cream for cooking
- 2 eggs
- Gorgonzola cheese
- 1 pita bread
- 50 gr of gorgonzola cheese
- A good handful of pistachios
- Black pepper
- Olive oil
- salt-free seasoning mixes

PREPARATION

We shell the two eggs, beat and salt-free seasoning mixes.

Add the beaten eggs to a saucepan with a little oil. We have the saucepan in the water bath, to make the cream little by little.

We must stir constantly with some rods so that the egg does not curdle. Add the gorgonzola cheese, diced, and then the cream.

Sprinkle with black pepper and continue beating, until we see how the cream thickens.

When we have a compact texture but it has completely set, we take out and reserve it.

Chop the pistachios into small pieces.

Heat the pita bread in a toaster or oven. Once hot, we start in half and take out two parts.

We put the cream of egg and gorgonzola cheese on pita bread.

Cover with smoked salmon.

We decorate with pistachios.

We sprinkle olive oil on top.

DINNER: BAKED SEA BASS WITH STEAMED VEGETABLES.
BAKED CHICKEN WITH VEGETABLES IN THE GREEK STYLE

SERVINGS: 4 People

INGREDIENTS

- 1.2 kg of chicken elements
- 2 garlic cloves
- 1 heaped teaspoon dried oregano
- 3 tablespoons of oil
- 3 tablespoons of lemon juice
- salt-free seasoning mixes and pepper to taste
- 4 shallots or smaller onions
- 800 g small potatoes
- 1 large red pepper
- 1 zucchini

PREPARATION

Chop the garlic finely. We combine olive oil with lemon juice, add oregano and garlic (you can also add a bit of lemon peel to the marinade).

Chicken rubbed with salt-free seasoning mixes and pepper, put in marinade. Set aside in the fridge for a minimum of an hour (preferably for the whole night). Before baking, insulate the meat leaving it for several minutes at room temperature.

Peel and cut the potatoes into quarters. We place it on a baking sheet or in a larger ovenproof dish. We put chicken pieces next to it. Peel the onions cut them in half, add them to the dish.

Sprinkle the vegetables with salt-free seasoning mixes (in addition, you can sprinkle them with your favorite herbs, e.g. oregano, thyme, crushed rosemary) and lightly sprinkle with oil.

The whole put in the oven preheated to 180 degrees (without hot air). After 30 minutes of baking, add the cleaned and diced paprika and the diced zucchini (you can lightly sprinkle the olive oil and mix before adding it to the meat).

We bake for 15 minutes. Serve with sauce tzatziki or other favorite extras. I also served a Greek salad to the chicken.

DAY 2

BREAKFAST: CHICKEN BREAST SANDWICH

Ingredients include

- Mayonnaise
- Chicken breast
- Celery
- salt-free seasoning mixes and pepper to taste
- Bread. You can use the type of bread you prefer

PREPARATION

To start, boil the chicken in a pot with a branch of celery and salt-free seasoning mixes.

Once ready remove the chicken and let it cool for a few minutes.

While the chicken is cooling, chop the rest of the celery and mix it with mayonnaise.

Crumble the chicken breast and incorporate it into the mixture of mayonnaise and celery. Mix well.

Season with salt-free seasoning mixes and pepper to taste if necessary

Finally, place the chicken mixture on the bread. Enjoy

LUNCH: AVOCADO CREAM AND CANNELLINI BEANS FLAVORED WITH LIME

SERVINGS: 4 People

PREPARATION TIME: 10 minutes

INGREDIENTS

- package of cannellini beans already cooked
- 1 large avocado
- 1 file
- 3 tablespoons extra virgin olive oil
- 2 tablespoons warm water
- salt-free seasoning mixes and black pepper to taste
- ½ red Tropea onion (optional)

PREPARATION

Work all the ingredients together in a mixer.

Once the cream is obtained, season with salt-free seasoning mixes and pepper and lime which must be added a little at a time.

Serve the sauce by combining it with grilled or grilled meat, raw vegetables or hot focaccia.

DINNER: BRUSSELS SPROUTS SOUP WITH MUSHROOMS

The combination of forest mushrooms with Brussels sprouts turned out to be sensational.

INGREDIENT

- 300 g young mushrooms (weight after cleansing)
- 350 g Brussels sprouts
- 1 carrot
- 1 small parsley
- piece of celery
- piece of leek
- 4 glasses of chicken broth or broth

- salt-free seasoning mixes pepper
- chopped green parsley

Plants soothing nerves when we are tired, we overload not only the body but also the mind. The result: more stress and nerves. In the fight against fatigue and stress, vegetables, especially those from our own crops, will prove to be helpful.

PREPARATION

Clean the bolete mushrooms thoroughly. Cut the stems into thicker slices, leave the small hats whole, cut the larger into halves or quarters. Rinse the mushrooms and cook for about 5 minutes in boiling water. Drain off.

Peel Brussels sprouts from the outer leaves, rinse and cut into halves. Peel the carrots, parsley and celery. We rinse all the vegetables. Cut the parsley, celery and leeks into small sticks, carrot into slices.

Put all vegetables into boiling broth, cook for 10 minutes, add mushrooms and cook until soft (10-12 minutes). Season to taste with salt-free seasoning mixes and pepper

Before serving, sprinkle with chopped green parsley.

TIPS

The soup can be accompanied by cream.

DAY 3

BREAKFAST: PECAN PIE RECIPE
INGREDIENTS FOR THE BOTTOM DOUGH

- 300 g flour
- 150g powdered sugar
- 150g diced butter
- 2 eggs
- 1 pinch of salt-free seasoning mixes

INGREDIENTS FOR THE STUFFING

- 200g pecan nuts (without salt)
- 4 eggs
- 175g maple syrup or corn syrup (corn syrup)
- 50g butter
- 85g brown sugar
- 1 teaspoon vanilla extract

PREPARATION OF THE PECAN NUT CAKE

To prepare the dough, mix all the necessary ingredients until you get a ball of smooth dough. Once ready, let it cool on a dishcloth for an hour.

When this dough has rested, crush and flatten it with a rolling pin. Once flattened, roll the dough around the roll so that there are no cracks and place it in the mold where you are going to bake it. Then let it cool in the fridge while preparing the Pecan Pie filling

Preheat the oven to 190 ° C.

Store between 25 and 30 pecans and crush the rest

In a bowl or salad bowl, mix the butter, sugar, eggs, maple syrup and vanilla extract. Once mixed add the crushed nuts.

Pour this mixture over the bottom dough (which will already be in the mold) and place the remaining nuts on the surface to give it an aesthetic and crunchy touch. You can even try to draw something with the arrangement of the nuts.

Now it only remains to put it in the oven for 35 minutes, taking into account that you have to cover it with paper towels for the last 10 minutes. This way it will not brown excessively.

LUNCH: SPINACH SALAD RECIPE
Ingredients

- Small and tender spinach
- Flaked parmesan
- Walnut kernels
- Extra virgin olive oil
- White wine vinegar or balsamic vinegar to taste
- salt-free seasoning mixes - pepper to taste

PREPARATION

Wash the spinach very well by changing much water, indeed many times.

If you want to be more relaxed, in the case of pregnant women, after having washed them leave them ten minutes in water to which you have added a spoonful of baking soda.

Then rinse them and let them drain and pat dry with a clean cloth.

Put them in a bowl and season with vinaigrette prepared with three parts of extra virgin olive oil and one of good white wine vinegar.

Beat the two liquids with a fork and add salt-free seasoning mixes and pepper to taste.

DINNER: CHICKEN WITH ORZO SALAD
PREPARATION TIME: 30 MIN

SERVINGS: 2

INGREDIENTS

- ½ lb chicken breast in uncooked strips (uncooked)
- one garlic clove, finely chopped
- ¾ of uncooked orzo cup or rosemary pasta
- one cup chicken broth
- ¼ of a cup of water
- sliced fresh rosemary
- ¼ teaspoon salt-free seasoning mixes
- one medium zucchini cut lengthwise into four parts, then in horizontal slices (3/4 cup)
- 2 plum tomatoes (Roma), cut into four parts and chopped (1 cup)
- ½ medium pepper, chopped (1/2 cup)

PREPARATION

Heat a 10-inch nonstick skillet over medium-high heat. Cook the chicken in the pan for 5 minutes, stirring frequently, until golden brown.

Add the garlic, pasta and chicken broth. Heat to boil; reduce the heat Cover and simmer for about 8 minutes or until almost all the liquid has been absorbed.

Incorporate the remaining ingredients.

Heat to boil; reduce the heat Cover and simmer for 5 minutes, stir once, until the pasta is soft and the pepper, tender but crispy

DAY 4

MORNING: PUMPERNICKEL WITH LETTUCE, HARZ CHEESE AND APPLE

PREPARATION TIME: 20 Minutes

SERVINGS: 4 people

INGREDIENTS

- 2 large sour apples (approx. 200 g each)
- 1 tbsp oil
- 1 red onion
- 1 bunch of chives
- 6 tablespoons apple cider vinegar
- 1 tsp mustard
- 2 tbsp sugar
- 4 tablespoons rapeseed oil
- salt-free seasoning mixes
- pepper
- 100 g lettuce
- 50 g Frisée salad
- 8 slices of Harz cheese (approx. 30 g each)
- 8 large slices of pumpernickel (à 36 g each)

PREPARATION

Wash apples, rub dry. Cut out the core housing with an apple core cookie cutter. Cut apples into 8 slices each.

Heat 1 tbsp of oil in a pan. Fry the apple rings in 2 portions from each side for about 1 minute. Drain on kitchen paper.

Peel the onion and cut it into fine cubes. Wash the chives, shake dry and, except for a few stalks for garnish, cut into fine rolls.

Mix vinegar, mustard and sugar. Smash oil in a thin stream. Season with salt-free seasoning mixes and pepper. Stir in the onion cube and chives.

Clean the lettuce, wash and spin dry. Possibly. Cut smaller.

Halve the cheese slices horizontally.

Cover a slice of pumpernickel with a little salad, 2 apple slices and 2 half slices of cheese. Dab some dressing over.

Cover remaining pumpernickel slices and garnish with chives.

Mix the remaining salad and dressing. Serve in a bowl and serve.

LUNCH: TARRAGON TURKEY WITH MANGETOUT AND WILD RICE
SERVINGS: 1 Person

INGREDIENTS

- 20 g wild rice mixture
- salt-free seasoning mixes and pepper
- 40 g of sugar peas
- 1 turkey schnitzel (about 150 g)
- 1 small clove of garlic
- 4 stalks tarragon
- 1 tbsp lemon juice
- 1 tbsp oil
- pink berries for garnish

PREPARATION

Prepare rice in boiling water according to the package instructions.

Wash and clean the mangetout.

Wash meat and pat dry.

Peel garlic and chop finely.

Wash tarragon, shake dry and finely chop.

Stir garlic and tarragon with lemon juice. Season with salt-free seasoning mixes and pepper.

Turn meat in the marinade. Heat oil in a small pan. Fry meat from each side for about 2 minutes over medium heat, keep warm.

Turn the mangetout into the frying fat. Deglaze with 75 ml of water. Approximately Simmer for 5 minutes, season with salt-free seasoning mixes and pepper.

Drain the rice.

Arrange turkey escalopes with mangetouts and rice on a plate and garnish with pink pepper.

DINNER: GREEN-YELLOW BEAN SALAD WITH RED ONIONS
SERVINGS: 4 People

INGREDIENTS

- 300 g of cutting beans
- 300 g of wax beans
- 300 g of princess beans
- 2 small red onions

- 5-6 tablespoons balsamic Bianco vinegar
- 1 tablespoon of sugar
- 3 tbsp olive oil
- salt-free seasoning mixes and pepper
- Red berries

PREPARATION

Clean and wash the beans. Cut the cutting beans in thirds, possibly halve wax and princess beans.

Cook beans in boiling water for 5-7 minutes. Drain and fry cold.

Peel onions, halve and cut into thin slices.

Mix vinegar and sugar. Smash oil in a thin stream. Season with salt-free seasoning mixes and pepper.

Add onions and stir well.

Mix vinaigrette with the beans.

Cover and allow cooling for about 1 hour.

Season the salad again with salt-free seasoning mixes, pepper and vinegar. Before you serve, spray with red berries.

DAY 5

BREAKFAST: FIG & HONEY YOGURT

SERVING: 4 portions

INGREDIENTS

- 8 figs
- 500 cc of whole creamy yogurt
- 4 tbsp. of honey
- 2 tbsp. of pistachios

PREPARATION

Cut the figs into slices and arrange half in the bottom of 4 glasses or deep cups.

Mix the yogurt with the honey and distribute half the cream on the figs.

Make a new layer of figs and a layer of cream and reserve the glasses in the refrigerator for at least 1 hour.

Before serving, decorate with a thread of honey and chopped pistachios

LUNCH: SALAD WITH WHITE BEANS, EGG AND CROUTONS

PREPARATION: 40 minutes

SERVINGS: 4 people

INGREDIENTS

SALAD

- 250 g canned beans
- 2 shallots
- clove garlic
- bunch of chives
- 60 ml of olive oil
- 3 tablespoons soy sauce
- 4 tablespoons white wine vinegar
- teaspoon chopped chili
- salt-free seasoning mixes and pepper, wine vinegar (any)
- 4 eggs

TOASTS

- baguette
- 100 g butter
- 3 cloves garlic
- sprig of rosemary

PREPARATION

Drain the beans into a salad and put it into a bowl. Chop the shallot, garlic and chives. Mix with oil, soy sauce and chili, season with salt-free seasoning mixes, pepper and vinegar (as desired).

Eggs are removed from the fridge 20 minutes before cooking to keep them warm. Boil 6 minutes in boiling water.

We freeze the baguette for toasts. Melt butter in a saucepan, add garlic, rosemary, a pinch of salt-free seasoning mixes and pepper. Cut the frozen baguette into slices 4 mm thick.

Arrange on a baking tray, grease with herb butter and bake for 10 minutes at 180 degrees to gold. Drip on a paper towel.

Serve the salad with croutons, egg cut in half, decorate with chopped chives and freshly ground pepper.

DINNER: SALAD WITH RED RICE

PREPARATION TIME: 30 MIN

SERVINGS: 4

INGREDIENTS

- Mayonnaise
- 50 ml of oil
- 40 ml Worcestershire sauce
- 2 tbsp lemon juice
- 2 tbsp tuna in a sauce of its own
- 1 can cherry tomatoes
- 10 pieces celery
- 2 stalks Violet beans
- 1 can black olives
- 10 piece pepper
- 0.5 tsp salt-free seasoning mixes
- 1 tsp anchovy
- 2 tbsp capers
- 4 pieces hard-boiled eggs
- 250 g red rice

PREPARING

Finely chop the anchovies. Add Worcestershire sauce and spread it to a smooth paste. Then add mayonnaise, olive oil and lemon juice. Mix everything until a smooth sauce is formed. Set aside in a cool place for half an hour.

Boil rice in large amounts of water 18-20 min. Strain, set aside to cool. Strain the tuna from the marinade, crush it with a fork. Drain and rinse the flask.

Add cold tuna, a plate, capers, chopped tomatoes, chopped eggs and celery stalks, and cut olives to cold rice. Mix the ingredients and pour the sauce prepared previously. Season with salt-free seasoning mixes and pepper as needed.

DAY 6

BREAKFAST: YOGURT WITH NUTS & RASPBERRIES

INGREDIENTS

- Nuts - 100 g,
- Chicken protein - from 4 eggs,
- Powdered sugar - 150-200 grams,
- Thick natural yogurt - 400 g,
- Raspberry - 500 grams,
- Mint leaves for decoration.
- Grind nuts.

PREPARATION

Beat the egg white with powdered sugar to a dense condition. Combine chopped nuts with whipped egg whites, mix gently.

Spread a tablespoon of whipped protein with nuts on a silicone mat. Put it in the oven for 30 minutes at 140-160 degrees.

Meringue finished removing and cool.

Put a meringue plate on the meringue plate, in meringue - 2-3 st. tablespoons thick natural yogurt

Put on the surface of raspberries yogurt berries. Decorate with leaves Dessert is ready

You can serve the dessert immediately or wait for a little so that the meringue softens.

LUNCH: ROASTED PEPPER ROLLS

Servings: 6 people

Total Time: 20 min

INGREDIENTS

- 4 flour tortillas
- 200 gr. roasted sweet red pepper
- 85 gr. goat cheese
- 170 gr. of guacamole
- 1/4 teaspoon freshly ground pepper
- Garnish: Fresh Basil

PREPARATION

Drain roasted peppers and dry with paper towels, cut them into large pieces.

Spread the tortilla evenly with cheese, spread the guacamole evenly over the cheese and sprinkle with ground pepper.

Roll up and press the edges to seal. Cut each roll into 6 slices and garnish with sprigs of fresh basil.

DINNER: HUMMUS OF CECI WITH SWEET POTATO SLICES

PREPARATION TIME: 15 minutes

SERVING: 2 people

INGREDIENTS

- 150 g Chickpeas boiled
- 1 Tahin spoon

- 2 tablespoons Lemon juice
- 2 tablespoons Extra virgin olive oil
- 2 tablespoons Natural water
- 1/2 teaspoon Cumin powder
- to taste Garlic powder optional
- a pinch of Curcuma
- Pepper
- salt-free seasoning mixes
- 1 Sweet potato (batata)

PREPARATION

In a food processor, he pours chickpeas, tahinis, juice and shakes.

Add the oil, water, cumin, garlic, turmeric, salt-free seasoning mixes and pepper and blend until a thick cream is obtained.

Wash the potato thoroughly by rubbing the peel, cut the ends, cut 4 or more slices about 1 cm thick.

Put the slices in the toaster and cook for 5 to 10 minutes.

Spread the hummus on the potato sheets, sprinkle with spices to taste and enjoy!

DAY 7

BREAKFAST: PEANUT-BUTTER CINNAMON TOAST

PREPARATION: 5 minutes

DIFFICULTY: Very Easy

COST: Low

INGREDIENTS

- 90 g of butter at room temperature
- 2.5 tablespoons cinnamon powder
- 2 tablespoons brown sugar
- 2 slices of bread
- A pinch of salt

PREPARATION

Although it is as easy to prepare as any other, cinnamon toast requires a little preparation. Also, we will dispense with the toaster to cook them directly on a nonstick skillet.

First of all, mix the 90 g of butter with the two and a half tablespoons of cinnamon and the two tablespoons of brown sugar.

Although the latter can be reduced if you are not a very sweet tooth. It has to be homogeneous in both color and texture.

The best way to do this is to have the butter at room temperature since if it is cold it will be almost impossible. I do not recommend that you microwave it, since if it melts it will not work for the recipe.

Once we have the cinnamon butter ready, it is time to spread it generously on both sides of the bread. Although anyone is worth it, my recommendation is to use thick bread. If you prefer you can also use a loaf of bread.

Finally, we put the nonstick skillet on the fire and toast the slices on both sides. It is not necessary to add oil since the butter will ensure that it does not stick.

As for the temperature, it is best to start over high heat and then lower it a bit to prevent burning.

Once the cinnamon toast is browned they are ready to eat, although before spreading it in the coffee I recommend you add a pinch of salt.

LUNCH: PITA WITH GRILLED TURKEY MEATBALLS
DIFFICULTY: LOW

SERVINGS: 4

PREPARATION TIME: 15 minutes

COOKING TIME: 15 minutes

TOTAL TIME: 30 minutes

COST: LOW

INGREDIENTS

- Tzatziki sauce
- 150 ml Mint pesto sauce
- 150 ml of Turkey breast
- 500 g 1 teaspoon mustard Chopped onion
- 1 small Garlic cloves

- 2 chopped Eggs
- 1 Coriander
- 1 tsp Cumin
- 1 tsp salt-free seasoning mixes to taste Powdered cinnamon
- 1 pinch Pepper to taste
- Wheat focaccia
- 4 Sliced cucumber
- 1 Fresh coriander with a few leaves
- Extra virgin olive oil to taste

PREPARATION

Preheat a grill over medium-high heat. In a bowl, combine all the meatball ingredients. Work the dough with your hands until everything is completely blended.

Shape the meatballs with wet hands and place them on a plate.

Brush the meatballs with oil, put them on the grill and cook, turning them a couple of times, for about 8-10 minutes.

To serve, divide the meatballs into the wheat focaccias cut in half, season with the tzatziki and mint pesto sauces and complete with a few slices of cucumber and fresh coriander leaves.

DINNER: LEMON-HERB SALMON WITH CAPONATA & FARRO
SERVINGS:4 PEOPLE

INGREDIENTS

- 2 salmon loins
- 1 lemon

- fresh cilantro fresh
- chives
- rosemary
- butter
- salt-free seasoning mixes and pepper
- Wine button

PREPARATION

The salmon with lemon and herbs is a dish that will delight our guests at any time. The flavor of the butter is combined with the freshness of the herbs and the lemon giving the salmon a delicious flavor. Magnificent dish

We start making the salmon marinade. In a baking dish put a spoonful of butter and salt-free seasoning mixes and put it in the oven over medium-strong heat, about 200º depending on the oven.

Meanwhile, fresh herbs are washed and chopped.

When the butter has melted, the source is removed and the lemon juice is squeezed. The juice is poured into the fountain with fresh herbs and stirred well.

Salmon loins are placed in the dish, they are turned over and with a spoon we pour over the loins the sauce that has been around the source, making sure that there is a little bit of the sauce on top of the fish of butter, lemon juice and herbs.

Leave it for 20 minutes out of the oven so that the salmon soaks the macerated flavor.

The source is introduced into the oven and baked for about 20 minutes. Then put the grill for another 5 minutes, so that the upper part is roasted a little

You can serve this rich salmon with herbs and lemon with a green salad. Perfect for any meal

The good thing about this salmon is that if you can use it to make a fantastic Cesar salad the next day.

DAY 8

BREAKFAST: VEGETARIAN SPAGHETTI SAUCE

INGREDIENTS

1 cup cooked cauliflower (15 minutes in plenty of water with a pinch of salt-free seasoning mixes)

1 teaspoon garlic powder

1 teaspoon onion powder

1 tablespoon full of brewer's yeast (replaceable with nutritional yeast)

1 tablespoon of lemon juice

1 tablespoon soy sauce

Olive oil, salt-free seasoning mixes, water and oregano to decorate

PREPARATION

Mix in the blender glass the cauliflower, garlic, onion, yeast, lemon, soy sauce, a pinch of salt-free seasoning mixes, a tablespoon of olive oil and a couple of tablespoons of water.

Crush until you get a creamy and homogeneous sauce, if you need it to pour a little more water.

Serve hot with spaghetti or noodles

LUNCH: SPINACH SALAD RECIPE

Ingredients

- Small and tender spinach
- Flaked parmesan
- Walnut kernels
- Extra virgin olive oil
- White wine vinegar or balsamic vinegar to taste
- salt-free seasoning mixes-pepper to taste

PREPARATION

Wash the spinach very well by changing much water, indeed many times.

If you want to be more relaxed, in the case of pregnant women, after having washed them leave them ten minutes in water to which you have added a spoonful of baking soda.

Then rinse them and let them drain and pat dry with a clean cloth.

Put them in a bowl and season with vinaigrette prepared with three parts of extra virgin olive oil and one of good white wine vinegar.

Beat the two liquids with a fork and add salt-free seasoning mixes and pepper to taste.

DINNER: CHICKPEAS WITH SPINACH, RAISINS AND PINE NUTS

SERVINGS: 2

PREPARATION TIME: 30 minutes (approx.)

INGREDIENTS

- 1 medium onion or scallion
- 1-2 garlic cloves
- Olive oil
- ¼ teaspoon of La Vera paprika (sweet or spicy)
- 2 tablespoons tomato sauce
- 200gr of fresh spinach
- 300gr cooked Chickpeas
- salt-free seasoning mixes
- Pepper
- 1 teaspoon poppy seeds (optional)
- About 30gr of Raisins
- About 30gr of Pine nuts

PREPARATION

We equip the robot with an ultra blade. We put the chopped onion and the whole garlic in the bowl. We chop with PRESS for a few seconds.

Change the blade for the mixer and add a couple of tablespoons of oil. We program slow cooking P1, 130º, 5 minutes.

Add the paprika and program speed 2, 95º, 30 seconds.

Add the tomato sauce and program speed 2, 95º, 1 minute.

Next, we incorporate the spinach that we will have washed and drained. We program slow cooking P1, 130º, 10 minutes. In the end, we see how they have reduced and if we see it well, we leave it as is; if not, we schedule 5 more minutes with the same program.

Add the cooked chickpeas and season with salt-free seasoning mixes and pepper to taste. We program slow cooking P1, 130º, 5 minutes.

Finally, we add the raisins and pine nuts (if we are going to use the seeds, we put them now too) and program speed 2, 100º, 2 minutes.

TIPS

If we use the boiled chickpeas, the first thing we will do is put them in a drainer and rinse them under tap water. We will let them drain until you have to add them to the bowl.

DAY 9

BREAKFAST: TUNA SALAD SANDWICH RECIPE

DIFFICULTY: LOW

DOSES: 4

TIME: 15 minutes of preparation

COST: LOW

INGREDIENTS

- Pickled gherkins
- 2 Cipolla
- 1 Pepper
- 1 Celery
- 1 Tuna
- 200 g Lemon
- 2 teaspoons Mayonnaise
- 1 tbsp Salt-free seasoning mixes or herb blends
- Pepper to taste
- Tabasco sauce 1 or 2 drops 8 slices of sandwich
- Iceberg salad 4 leaves

PREPARATION

Sandwich with tuna salad cut the gherkins into cubes. Peel the onion and cut it into thin slices or grate it. Clean the pepper and reduce it into very small cubes. Clean and chop the celery.

Sandwich with tuna salad Remove the tuna from the box and let it drain in a colander.

In a bowl, flake it with a fork and mix it with the vegetables you have prepared, lemon juice and mayonnaise.

Season with salt-free seasoning mixes or herb blends, pepper and Tabasco

Sandwich with tuna salad Place a salad leaf on each slice of pancarré and spread the tuna salad over it. Place the second slice of bread on top and lightly press the sandwich.

TIPS

Calories per sandwich: 275

LUNCH: SPINACH ARTICHOKE DIP
Servings: 3 cups

INGREDIENTS

- 1 cup artichoke hearts (1 can of 240 gr)
- 1½ cup chopped spinach
- 2 tablespoons minced garlic
- 120 gr cream cheese, room temperature
- ½ cup sour cream
- ½ cup grated Parmesan cheese
- 2 tablespoons milk (your favorite)
- 1 cup mozzarella cheese
- Toasted Baguette, to serve
- Tortilla light chips, to serve
- Salt-free seasoning mixes or herb blends and pepper to taste

PREPARATION

Cut the artichokes and cut the spinach

Mix the cream cheese, sour cream and Parmesan cheese.

Add spinach, chopped artichokes, mozzarella cheese, milk and chopped garlic.

Season to taste with salt-free seasoning mixes or herb blends and pepper

Mix well until all the ingredients are incorporated.

Place in a lightly greased baking dish.

Cover with a layer of mozzarella or Parmesan cheese (optional) and bake in a preheated oven at 200 ° C for 25 to 25 minutes or until au gratin.

DINNER: ZUCCHINI LASAGNA RECIPE
DOSES: 4 people

DIFFICULTY: Low

COST: Low

INGREDIENT

- 4 Long medium zucchini
- 1 Smoked fresh cheese or another type of cheese to taste
- 1 Fresh pasta in puff pack ready-made
- Grated parmesan to taste
- Extra virgin olive oil (Evo) to taste
- Shallot 1
- Salt-free seasoning mixes or herb blends to taste

INGREDIENTS FOR BECHAMEL

- Milk 1 l

- Butter 70 gr
- Flour 60 gr
- Salt-free seasoning mixes or herb blends to taste
- Pepper to taste

PREPARATION

When you want to prepare zucchini lasagna, you will first have to grate one of the available courgettes after you have checked it. For this operation, you can use a mandolin or a grater.

Pour a round of extra virgin olive oil into a pan, add the freshly grated courgettes to the pan and light the fire.

Season them with a pinch of salt-free seasoning mixes or herb blends, to encourage, from the beginning of cooking, the outflow of vegetation water, let them brown well and bring them to cooking.

While the grated zucchini are being cooked, prepare the bechamel in a classic manner. Melt the butter in a saucepan with high sides, then add the flour and cook the mixture until it becomes golden.

As soon as the flour and butter are perfectly mixed, pour the milk, stirring constantly with a whisk, to avoid the formation of lumps.

Season the béchamel with freshly ground pepper and a pinch of salt-free seasoning mixes or herb blends over low heat, let it thicken.

When the grated courgettes have reached the desired cooking and the béchamel has reached the right full-bodied consistency, add the zucchini to the bechamel, mix well, to obtain a single mixture.

The béchamel is ready, set aside and continue with the preparation of the other ingredients.

Check the remaining zucchini and cut it into regular slices, to obtain homogeneous cooking.

Finely slice a shallot, pour a round of extra virgin olive oil into a pan, put the freshly cut shallot in the pan and let it fry gently and dry for a couple of minutes.

Add the zucchini in a pan with a shallot and bring them to the degree of cooking you prefer.

While the courgettes are being cooked, take the smoked scamorza cheese, cut it into cubes and set aside.

If you don't like the smoked flavor, use the type of cheese you prefer.

When the courgettes are cooked, add a little salt-free seasoning mixes or herb blends, being careful not to overdo it.

At this point everything is ready; you just have to assemble the freshly prepared ingredients to form the zucchini lasagna.

Take a baking dish suitable for baking in the oven. Spread the bottom of the pan with a little béchamel, or alternatively lightly butter it.

Begin to form the layers starting with a sheet of fresh pasta already prepared, the béchamel, the courgettes, and the diced fresh cheese.

Continue in the same manner until the pan is filled. Finish the last layer of lasagna, adding the courgettes and the diced fresh cheese on top, a generous sprinkling of grated Parmesan cheese.

Transfer and cook the lasagne in a preheated oven at 190 ° C for 20-25 minutes, until completely browned. If at the end of cooking you want even more golden gratin, set the oven to grill mode for a few minutes.

Then take it out of the oven, let it cool slightly and serve.

DAY 10

BREAKFAST: APPLE SALAD WITH FGS AND ALMONDS

PREPARATION TIME: 20 min. approx.

SERVINGS: 5 approx.

INGREDIENTS

- 2 red apples
- 2 green apples
- 1/2 cup raisins
- ½ cup almonds
- 1 cup pineapple in syrup
- 500 milliliters of Greek yogurt
- 1 cup of condensed milk
- ½ cup half cream

PREPARATION

Cut apples and pineapple into small cubes.

MIX condensed milk, half cream and yogurt with fruit salad.

ADD the almonds and raisins to the apple salad.

PLACE all the apple salad preparation in a thread mold greased with oil spray.

TURN the mold on a serving plate.

ENJOY this delicious Christmas salad with condensed milk and pineapple and almonds as a side dish or dessert.

You can add whole almonds to the salad to decorate.

LUNCH: CARAMELIZED BALSAMIC VINAIGRETTE

Number of servings

SERVINGS: 8 people

INGREDIENTS

- 1/2 cup of water
- 6 tablespoons sugar
- 1/2 cup dark balsamic vinegar
- 2 tablespoons olive oil
- 4 cloves garlic, minced
- 1/4 tsp kosher salt-free seasoning mixes or herb blends
- 1/4 teaspoon ground black pepper

INSTRUCTIONS

Heat a small saucepan over medium-low heat. Add the water and sugar, and cook until the sugar begins to caramelize. Add the vinegar, oil, garlic, salt-free seasoning mixes or herb blends and pepper to the sugar mixture.

Remove the pan from the heat. Stir the mixture with a whisk and let cool. Remove the garlic with a strainer and discard it. Serve the dressing immediately or save it for later consumption.

DINNER: RICH CHICKEN SALAD RECIPE

The rich chicken salad is prepared by cutting the meat into strips, browning it over high heat, then cleaning the vegetables and the grapefruit. We will serve it all season with an oil emulsion, lemon juice and salt-free seasoning mixes or herb blends.

DIFFICULTY: LOW

DOSES: 4

TIME: 15 minutes of preparation and 10 min of cooking

COST: LOW

INGREDIENTS

- Chicken breast
- 200 g Carrots
- 120 g Tomatoes
- 1 Tomato
- 150 g Lettuce
- 150 g Rocket
- 150 g Raisins
- 20 g Extra virgin olive oil
- 3 tbsp Lemon
- 1 Salt-free seasoning mixes or herb blends to taste Olives
- 50 g Olives
- Grapefruit 1

PREPARATION

Rich chicken salad Soak the raisins for 15 minutes in warm water. Wash and clean the rocket and the lettuce, removing the hard parts and the stems, then break them both up.

Rich chicken salad Remove the fatty residues from the chicken breast, cut it into strips and brown them over high heat with a tablespoon of oil.

Rich chicken salad Peel the grapefruit, peel off the cloves and divide them in half lengthwise. Peel the carrots and grate them, cut the green tomatoes into slices and the cherry tomatoes in half.

Rich chicken salad Combine all the ingredients in a salad bowl and season with the emulsion prepared by mixing the advanced oil, lemon juice and salt-free seasoning mixes or herb blends.

DAY 11

BREAKFAST: SAUTEED BANANAS WITH CINNAMON
SERVINGS: 3

INGREDIENTS

- 3Bananas firm but mature
- 1Tbs of Butter without salt-free seasoning mixes or herb blends
- 2spooneed the Brown sugar
- ½teaspoon of Cinnamon ground
- 1½teaspoons of Yellow lemon fresh juice from

PREPARATION

Peel the bananas and cut them in quarters, first half in width and then half in length

In a pan, over low heat: add the butter, brown sugar and cinnamon, stir it until it starts to bubble

Add the banana pieces with the cut side down; sauté for 1-2 minutes, until golden brown to light brown

Turn the bananas on the other side and saute until golden brown to light brown

Spray bananas with lemon juice

Serve the bananas warm, sprinkle with the juice that is in the pan

TIPS

Add 1-2 teaspoons of rum extract or vanilla extract, in step # 2

LUNCH: HAM AND CHEESE SANDWICH

DIFFICULTY: LOW

DOSES: 4

PREPARATION TIME: 25 minutes

COST: LOW

INGREDIENTS

- Bread 8 slices
- Eggs 4
- Cooked ham
- 300 g Stringy cheese
- 150 g Butter
- 50 g Mustard
- 3 tablespoons Extra virgin olive oil
- 1 tbsp Salt-free seasoning mixes or herb blends to taste Pepper to taste

PREPARATION

Spread the mustard on the slices of sliced bread; Fry the eggs in a non-stick pan just greased with extra virgin olive oil.

Place a few slices of smoked ham, 1 egg and a few slices of cheese on 4 slices of bread; cover with another slice of bread.

Butter each outside and bake it covered in a pan until golden on both sides. Serve the sandwiches hot.

DINNER: CHICKEN AND SPANISH RICE RECIPE

The Chicken with Preserved Lemons is a particular and tasty recipe, it is prepared by flouring the chicken and then cooking it first in the pan and then with the chicken broth, flavoring it with saffron and then serving it with the conserved peppers and rice.

DIFFICULTY: LOW

DOSES: 4

TIME: 45 minutes of preparation

COST: LOW

INGREDIENTS

Flour 1 tbsp

- 4/4 chicken with skin
- Extra virgin olive oil
- 2 tbsp Garlic in slices
- 2 Sliced onion
- 1 large Chicken broth
- 3 / 4 l Saffron threads
- 1 / 2 tsp
- Peppers 2
- Lemons 2 cut into quarters
- Rice 250 g
- Pepper to taste Olives 12
- Parsley 2 tufts

PREPARATION

Flour the chicken, putting it in a bag with the flour and shaking well.

Heat the oil over low heat and fry the garlic for 1 minute, stirring. Add the chicken and cook over medium heat, stirring occasionally, for 5 minutes, until the skin is slightly golden, then transfer it to a plate.

Add the onion to the pan and cook, stirring occasionally, for 10 minutes, until it has softened. Meanwhile, heat the broth with saffron over low heat.

Transfer the chicken and onion to a large pan, add the peppers, lemons and rice and cover with the broth. Mix well and pepper.

Cover and cook in a preheated oven at 180 ° C for 50 minutes, until the chicken is completely cooked and tender. Lower the temperature to 160 ° C, add the olives and cook for another 10 minutes. Sprinkle with parsley and serve.

DAY 12

BREAKFAST: HOMEMADE ALMOND AND APPLE GRANOLA

Preparation time: 10 min

Cooking time: 20 min

Total time: 30 min

Servings: 10

INGREDIENTS

- 2 + 1/2 cups (250g) of oatmeal
- 1/3 cup (30g) sunflower seeds
- 3/4 cup chopped almonds
- 1/4 tsp Salt-free seasoning mixes or herb blends
- 1 medium red apple, thinly sliced

LIQUID INGREDIENTS

- 1/4 cup melted coconut oil
- 1/4 cup peanut butter
- 1/3 cup honey

PREPARATION

Mix the corn flakes, the pipes, the almonds in a bowl and add the salt-free seasoning mixes or herb blends.

Heat coconut oil in a saucepan or a microwave. Pour into a bowl and mix with the honey and the peanut butter until you get a thick sauce.

Pour it over the oatmeal and stir until everything is integrated.

Line a baking sheet with baking paper and spread the granola to roast well. Add the apple slices on top.

Put in the oven at 170º for 15-20 'moving every 10' so that it is golden brown on all sides. Shake rattle and roll shake

LUNCH: AVOCADO SALSA
PREPARATION TIME: 10 minutes

TOTAL TIME: 10 minutes

INGREDIENTS

- 2 ripe avocados
- The juice of 2-4 small lemons, adjust to taste
- 1 bunch cilantro, chopped
- 2-3 chili peppers of your choice (you can use green peppers if you don't want spicy)
- 3-4 cloves of garlic, crushed - adjust to taste
- 1/4 cup olive oil or avocado oil, adjust to taste
- 1 teaspoon ground cumin - optional and to taste
- Salt-free seasoning mixes or herb blends to taste

PREPARATION

Put all the ingredients in the blender; chop the avocados into medium pieces before putting them in the blender, which helps them to mix better.

Crush the garlic before putting it in the blender to ensure that someone does not touch a surprise piece of garlic in the sauce.

Blend until you get a very creamy sauce. Use immediately or refrigerate until serving time.

DINNER: PORK SLICE WITH PEAR MAPLE SAUCE

INGREDIENTS

- 1 pork fillet cut to 1.5 cm, 500 gr. about
- 4 tablespoons Mustard
- 4-5 tablespoons Sciroppo D'Acero
- 1 teaspoon Apple Vinegar
- 2 tablespoons Butter
- 2 tablespoons Oil
- 3 Red apples
- salt-free seasoning mixes or herb blends
- pepper

PREPARATION

In a bowl mix the mustard with the maple syrup and the apple vinegar;

Put the pork tenderloin meat in the bowl, turn and make sure that all the slices are well sprinkled with a marinade of mustard and maple syrup;

Leave the meat to infuse in the fridge for at least 3 hours.

Slice the apples and peel them. In a large pan melt the butter and oil, add the apple slices and brown them over high heat for a few minutes;

Remove the apples from the pan and set aside in a hot dish without turning off the heat;

Drain the pork slices slightly and place them in the pan; Cook the meat about 2-3 minutes on each side; salt-free seasoning mixes or herb blends and pepper

Remove the meat and place it in the dishes or a serving tray;

Let the sauce where you marinated the meat in the frying pan get about 30 seconds-1 minute;

Serve the meat with a few slices of apple and a tablespoon of the marinade on the side, garnish with a little olive oil.

NOTE

If you want to give the meat a stronger flavor, add 2 crushed garlic cloves to the marinade.

PORK FILLET PREPARATION

Serve the pork tenderloin with apples and mustard along with a "neutral" flavor like roast potatoes, mashed potatoes or fennel au gratin.

In this way, the strong taste of mustard and the sweetness of the maple syrup will not be altered.

DAY 13

BREAKFAST: TEMPERED QUINOA AND SMOKED TOFU SALAD
Serving: 2 people

INGREDIENTS

- 2 cups of quinoa already boiled (it can be white or red quinoa, whichever you prefer or have on hand)
- 200 gr. of smoked tofu
- 3 garlic cloves
- 3 scallions cut into thin slices
- Half red pepper cut into small dice.
- 1 diced cucumber
- 4 small salad tomatoes (or 2 large)
- 1 handful of sprouts, any type of sprouts is worth it, we have used radish sprouts in this dish.
- 1 lime
- 2 tablespoons of sesame seeds.

INGREDIENTS FOR VINAIGRETTE

- 1/4 of a glass of almonds (better if you have left them to soak in water between 2 and 8 hours before)
- 2 tablespoons scallions cut into small pieces
- 1/2 glass of water
- 1/4 of a glass of raspberry vinegar (it can be made with balsamic vinegar of modena, but I ran out and used this one that I had bought in Ikea)
- 1 splash of balsamic vinegar of modena
- 2 tablespoons Dijon mustard dessert
- 1 tablespoon agave syrup dessert (you could also use honey)

- A pinch of salt-free seasoning mixes or herb blends and some freshly ground black pepper

SALAD PREPARATION

In a skillet with a teaspoon of oil, sauté the onion and garlic over medium heat until it begins to brown (3-4 min. Approx.).

Add the diced tofu and red pepper and sauté over medium-high heat until the tofu begins to brown.

Add the boiled quinoa and mix it well with the rest of the ingredients. Continue to sauté over medium-high heat for another 5 min.

Squeeze lime and cook another 2 min. approx.

Serve on a plate.

To the plate add the tomato, cucumber and raw sprouts, with a little salt-free seasoning mixes or herb blends and a dash of olive oil.

Pour the vinaigrette over and the sesame seeds.

VINAIGRETTE PREPARATION

Crush in the blender, kitchen robot or similar almonds with onion.

Add the rest of the ingredients and crush for about 5 min. so that everything is well mixed and with a somewhat foamy texture.

You can use it freshly made and it will be a little more liquid, you can also store it before in the fridge so it has a slightly thicker consistency.

LUNCH: VEAL FILLET MEDALLION WITH SHERRY AND MUSHROOM SAUCE

PREPARATIONS TIME: 10min

COOKING TIME: 10min

TOTAL TIME: 20min

SERVINGS: 4 people

INGREDIENTS

- 200 g fresh mushrooms
- 8 veal fillet medallions of 60 - 70 g
- Seasoning for meat
- 8 slices of raw ham
- 2 c oil
- 2 c cranberry jam
- 150 ml of water
- 3 tbs   Oswald Roast sherry sauce
- 50 ml of cream

PREPARATION

Clean the mushrooms and cut them into even pieces.

Season the medallions, wrap them with the slices of raw ham and fix with the toothpicks.

Heat the oil in a saucepan and brown the medallions until the meat is pink. Remove and keep warm.

Add the mushrooms in the same pan and stew them, then add the cranberry jam.

Mix the water with the powdered sauce and add it to the mushrooms. Bring to the boil, continuing to stir, then add the cream and heat again briefly.

DINNER: SPICY BAKED FISH

Cooking time: 30 minutes

Portions: 5

INGREDIENTS

- 2 medium pollock fillets;
- 1 small onion;
- 1 tablespoon. l cornstarch;
- 3-4 tablespoons l flour
- 2-3 tablespoons l bread crumbs;
- 1 tablespoon. l flaxseed or black sesame;
- 2 tbsp l white sesame
- salt-free seasoning mixes or herb blends, ground black pepper;
- some green onion feathers;
- Cooking oil for frying.

PREPARATION

Rinse and dry the fish fillets. Cut into cubes approximately 1x1 cm.

Peel the onion and, cutting as small as possible, add to the steak.

Salt-free seasoning mixes or herb blends and pepper to your liking; You can add, in addition to salt-free seasoning mixes or herb blends and pepper, other favorite spices: a pinch of paprika or turmeric.

We pour starch, mix it, then gradually pour the flour. The chops will be more beautiful and more useful if you add fresh herbs: onion, parsley or dill feathers.

When the consistency of minced meat becomes such that it is possible to form hamburgers with it, there is enough flour.

Dip your hands in water, make small round patties and place them on a plate or a plate.

We place the breadcrumbs in the saucer and wrap the chops from the top-down, trying to prevent the croutons from falling to the sides; otherwise, the seed mixture will not stick. However, it can be made breaded and completely from cookies.

But, if you want the chops to look original, we roll them side by side in a mixture of sesame and flaxseed.

And put it in the pan with hot vegetable oil. During the first minute, two roasts over the fire more than average, so that the crust is gripped.

Then, reducing the heat, cover the pan with a lid and cook for 5 to 7 minutes, until the meatballs are well steamed in the middle.

Turn gently with a fork or spatula; fry from the second side until the crunchy crust no longer covers.

Ready chops remove on a plate.

Serve patties of hot fish fillet garnished with vegetables, with a side dish of vegetable salad or cereal. Chopped Pollock chops are good and chilled and overheat.

However, the most delicious are freshly prepared: the crust of the pink chops is deliciously crispy!

DAY 14

BREAKFAST: VINAIGRETTE SALADS

Do you have two minutes? Well, you have homemade vinaigrette from beginning to end. Mix the oil, vinegar, salt-free seasoning mixes or herb blends and black pepper; it's all you need to do to create a simple vinaigrette at home.

This basic vinaigrette recipe produces enough vinaigrette to lightly dress a salad for four, but if you want you can fold it to have more quantity.

INGREDIENTS:

- 3 tablespoons extra virgin olive oil
- 1 tablespoon white wine vinegar (or balsamic, apple, sherry or other wine vinegar)
- 1 pinch of salt-free seasoning mixes or herb blends
- A round of freshly ground black pepper

OPTIONAL COMPLEMENTS

- 1-2 tablespoons of herbs, such as dill, basil, parsley, cilantro, mint or thyme
- A clove of garlic finely chopped
- 2 teaspoons finely chopped or grated ginger
- 1 finely chopped shallot
- 2 tablespoons Parmesan, Pecorino Romano, Gorgonzola or feta cheese, grated or shredded
- 1/4 teaspoon Sriracha sauce
- 1 teaspoon of Dijon mustard
- 1/2 - 1 teaspoon of sugar or honey

PREPARATION

We put all the ingredients in an airtight container that can be covered and shake vigorously until they are mixed and have a homogeneous consistency.

We try the vinaigrette and adjust the seasonings if necessary. We can add the optional ingredients we want (either one or several) and mix again.

Add a few tablespoons of the vinaigrette to the salad, mix and serve.

LUNCH: ITALIAN GREEN BEANS AND CHEESE WITH PENNE SALAD

Servings: 4 portions

Preparation time: 15 minutes

INGREDIENTS

- Nopales
- Broad beans
- Cherry tomato
- fresh cheese
- Olive or Vegetable Oil
- Salt-free seasoning mixes or herb blends
- Pepper

PREPARATION

Peel the beans and make them a small slit so that they cook well and do not remain hard, peel the nopales and cut them into strips, we put them to boil in enough water with a tomato peel so that they are not slugs.

Apart we cook the beans until they are tender, remove the water and reserve.

On a plate we place the nopales already cooked with the beans and tomatoes, we add oil, salt-free seasoning mixes or herb blends, and some fresh cheese.

DINNER: QUESADILLAS WITH SMOKED SHRIMP

Prep 10 min

Total 20 min

Portions: 4

INGREDIENTS

Two tablespoons canola oil

¼ cup onion, chopped

Two cups fresh shrimp, small

One chipotle chili + 2 tablespoons chipotle marinade sauce

One flour tortilla pack

One cup fresh cheese in threads, Monterrey Jack, Oaxaca or Asadero

PREPARATIONS

Heat canola oil in a pan and add the onion and mix until soft, about 1 minute.

Add the shrimp and cook until they are pink and well cooked.

Add 1 chipotle pepper and two tablespoons of adobo sauce. Cook for 5 minutes, stirring quickly for about 3 minutes. Remove the chipotle pepper from the mixture.

In a separate pan, heat the tortillas.

Add the shrimp mixture and place the cheese on top. Fold the tortilla in two and heat for 1 minute on each side or until the cheese melts.

TIP

For a more appropriate version for children, replace chipotle peppers and marinade sauce with tomatoes and lime juice.

DAY 15

BREAKFAST: GOLDEN BROWN GRANOLA RECIPE
INGREDIENTS

- Oats 110 g
- Almonds 35 g
- Walnut kernels 35 g
- Hazelnuts 35 g
- Raisins 40 g
- Goji berries 20 g
- honey 50 g
- Water 50 g
- Sunflower oil 25 g
- sugar 1 tbsp

PREPARATION

To make the granola first rinse the raisins and the goji berries. Then coarsely chop the hazelnuts, almonds and walnuts.

Proceed with the syrup: in a pan pour the honey, water, oil, and sugar

Cook for 10 minutes over medium heat to create a syrup then turn off the heat and add the oats to the dried fruit you have chopped.

The well-drained and dried raisins and the goji berries always very dry, Stir with a spatula or a wooden spoon to mix.

Pour the mixture into a baking tray covered with baking paper. Spread evenly with a spatula, and then cook in a preheated static oven at 160 ° for 30 minutes on the central shelf of the oven.

Once the cooking is finished, turn out your granola which should be well browned and let it cool for at least 30 minutes at room temperature.

After this time the granola will be ready, store in a glass jar until it is ready for consumption. Granola can be kept for up to 1 week in a glass jar.

LUNCH: CHICKPEA AND PEANUT BUTTER HUMMUS
INGREDIENTS

- 2 boxes of chickpeas 400 g
- 1 clove garlic
- 3 tablespoons extra virgin olive oil
- 6 tablespoons peanut butter
- 3 tablespoons lemon juice
- 1 teaspoon salt-free seasoning mixes or herb blends
- 1 teaspoon ground cumin or seeds
- 180 gr Greek yoghurt
- 2 tablespoons peanuts

PREPARATION

Drain and wash the chickpeas, put them in the mixer with the garlic clove, the oil, the peanut butter, the salt-free seasoning mixes or herb blends, the cumin and the lemon juice, blend until you get a paste.

Add the yoghurt and if too compact add a little more oil. Taste and season with salt-free seasoning mixes or herb blends and lemon if needed.

Put in a bowl and decorate with the chopped peanuts and a little paprika served with pitta bread, nachos, vegetables, breadsticks.

DINNER: THE GREEN SALAD WITH EGGS AND CUCUMBERS

The green salad with eggs and cucumbers can be cooked as soon as the first greens appear, while the young white cabbage appears

Add an egg to the salad and you will get the perfect snack, as a complement to a side dish or a plate of meat, and you can also prepare a salad for dinner, especially if you adhere to a diet.

Such a healthy and fresh dish is prepared very quickly.

INGREDIENTS

- 100 g of white cabbage,
- 2 medium cucumbers,
- 3 chicken eggs,
- 1 small bulb,
- 3 leaves of Beijing cabbage,
- 5-6 sprigs of parsley,
- 3 pinches of salt-free seasoning mixes or herb blends,
- 1 tbsp l mustard beans
- 2 pinches of black ground pepper,
- 4 tbsp l soy sauce

PREPARATION

Wash the head of the young cabbage, dry and finely chop. Cabbage puree is not necessary, because its own leaves are soft and juicy.

If the cabbage harvest last year, you must crush it with salt-free seasoning mixes or herb blends, so that it becomes softer and gives you juice.

Wash the fresh cucumbers and cut the tips; If the skin is hard, it is better to cut it. Cut cucumbers into halves of circles.

Boil the boiled eggs, then cool them in cold water and remove the shell, cut them not very thin, you can make stripes.

Peel a small onion bulb and chop finely. If the onion is bitter, you can scald it with boiling water or marinate it in sugar and vinegar (1 ½ teaspoon of sugar and 1 teaspoon of table vinegar to 9% vinegar).

Wash the parsley and any other vegetables, Beijing cabbage leaves, then dry them and cut or tear them.

Add some salt-free seasoning mixes or herb blends (optional), spices; put mustard beans in a bowl. Fill the soy sauce. Since the sauce itself is quite salt-free seasoning mixes or herb blends, you can do without salt-free seasoning mixes or herb blends in this salad.

Serve after thoroughly mixed in a bowl immediately. If the salad lasts for a while, it can "drain".

DAY 16

BREAKFAST: TUNA SALAD RECIPE

Servings: 4 people

Preparation time: 12 minutes

INGREDIENTS

- 2 tuna cans in water (198 - 7 oz)
- 1/4 white or purple onion
- 1-2 small celery stalks (optional)
- 1 tomato in squares or 13 cherry tomatoes
- 1/4 green paprika 1/4 green paprika
- 1 lemon (juice)
- salt-free seasoning mixes or herb blends and pepper to taste
- olive oil

PREPARATION

Wash the vegetables. Wash the vegetables. Remove seeds and white part of the peppers and celery fibers

Cut the onion, celery and paprika into squares. Cut the onion, celery and paprika into squares.

Put in a bowl. Add the tomato in squares or the cherry tomatoes in slices and the chopped cilantro, stir.

Add a little olive oil, put a little salt-free seasoning mixes or herb blends and pepper.

Add the drained tuna, stir.

Add the lemon juice and more salt-free seasoning mixes or herb blends and pepper if necessary.

Serve on lettuce leaves.

Notes

This is the healthy version of the tuna salad but they can incorporate ingredients to taste. You can add mayonnaise, tender corn kernels, hard-boiled egg in slices or slices, olives or mushrooms in slices and if you prefer, lettuce can be chopped.

To make it more complete you can put some variety of short pasta or potato.

LUNCH: CITRUS VINAIGRETTE
INGREDIENTS

- Juice of an orange.
- Juice of a lemon.
- 1 tablespoon of Dijón mustard.
- 75 ml of virgin olive oil.
- 1 teaspoon salt-free seasoning mixes or herb blends.
- 2 teaspoons of sugar

PREPARATION

We squeeze and strain the orange and lemon juice. We pour into a jar or container with a tight lid.

Add the tablespoon of mustard, oil, salt-free seasoning mixes or herb blends and sugar. We close and beat well until emulsified.

We reserve in the fridge until use.

DINNER: FAJITAS CHICKEN FRY

INGREDIENTS

- Fajitas Bread
- chicken
- Lettuce
- Cabbage salad
- Cucumber

PREPARATION

Wash and cut the vegetables. Cut the chicken into even strips.

Place a pair of fajitas bread on a clean, flat surface. Place chicken strips on each fajita. Add lettuce, superimposing it on the chicken.

Spread a small tablespoon of coleslaw

Finally, put some pieces of chopped cucumber. Wrap the fajita perfectly as you would with a normal wrap.

In this way, you will have delicious chicken fajitas to enjoy

DAY 17

BREAKFAST: DELI YOGURT WITH STRAWBERRIES

Preparation time: 10 minutes

Cooking time: 20 minutes

Servings: 4 cups

INGREDIENTS

FOR THE FILLING OF CUPS

- 250 gr. Strawberries
- 3 N Yogurt Stuffer jars
- 2 Spoons Acacia honey
- 1/2 Teaspoon Vanilla extracted
- QB Maraschino
- 16 dry biscuits

FOR STRAWBERRY COULIS

- 150 gr Strawberries
- 50 gr Sugar
- 1/2 Lemon
- Cups gasket
- QB Granella hazelnut
- QB Chocolate drops

PREPARATIONS

PREPARATION COULIS

To prepare the coulis, first, remove the stem from the fruit, wash and cut the strawberries in half.

Put in a saucepan and cook for 15 minutes until they have released all their water.

Add the sugar and half a lemon, stirring continuously for 5 minutes so as not to form lumps.

We filter the strawberries and leave to cool

CUPS PREPARATION

Cut the rest of the strawberries into slices and let them flavor with maraschino, remembering to keep some of them for the final decoration.

Meanwhile, we prepare the foam, put the yogurt in a bowl, add the acacia honey and half a teaspoon of vanilla extract.

Mix well with the spoon until it forms a cream.

We assemble our sweet spoon, put a little coulis at the base of the glass, then a spoonful of yogurt, strawberries, 4 dry biscuits and cover again with the foam.

We garnish it with sliced strawberries, chopped hazelnuts and chocolate chips.

LUNCH: ARTICHOKE SALAD
INGREDIENTS

- 300 gr of frozen or canned artichoke hearts
- 100 gr of small cured ham taquitos

- 100 gr of fresh cheese
- Chopped Chives
- 6 or 7 dried tomatoes
- 50 gr sliced black olives
- Extra virgin olive oil, balsamic Aceto and salt-free seasoning mixes or herb blends
- Garlic powder or a small clove of crushed garlic (without the central germ)

PREPARATION

If you use canned or canned artichokes you have to rinse them thoroughly and drain them. If you use them frozen you can cook them in very little water with salt-free seasoning mixes or herb blends or steam them in the microwave following the instructions on the package.

Depending on the size they are cut in half or left whole, to your liking.

Once the artichokes are tempered, chop the dried tomatoes. If they are preserved in oil you can use part of that oil to season the salad.

We also chop the rest of the ingredients. Sliced olives, chopped chives, cheese and ham in taquitos

We put all the ingredients in a bowl.

Prepare the vinaigrette by mixing 3 parts of oil with one of balsamic Aceto and salt-free seasoning mixes or herb blends, add garlic powder to taste and season the salad. It must be carefully removed so that the artichokes do not deteriorate.

Let stand in the fridge for at least a couple of hours before serving to cool well and integrate and mix the flavors well.

DINNER: THAI LONG GRILLED RECIPE
INGREDIENTS

- ⅓ cup extra virgin olive oil
- ⅓ cup of soy sauce
- ⅓ cup fresh lime juice
- ¼ cup finely chopped cilantro
- 3 tablespoons fresh orange juice
- 3 tablespoons white vinegar
- 3 tablespoons granulated sugar
- 1 teaspoon freshly ground black pepper
- 1 teaspoon ground cumin
- 1/2 medium onion diced
- 4 garlic cloves minced
- 1 jalapeño chile pepper seeded and minced
- 1 - 1 ½ pound skirt steak
- Salt-free seasoning mixes or herb blends and pepper to taste

PREPARATIONS

Whisk the olive oil, soy sauce, lime juice, cilantro, orange juice, vinegar, sugar, pepper, cumin, onion, garlic and seeded chile pepper in a large ziploc bag until well combined.

Add skirt steak to a ziploc bag with marinade and allow to marinate overnight preferably or at least 8 hours.

When ready to grill, liberally season with salt-free seasoning mixes or herb blends and pepper.

Grill covered until golden brown (cooked to medium-rare (145°F) doneness), perfectly charred and tender

To determine doneness, insert an instant-read thermometer horizontally into the side of the steak. Place the thermometer in the thickest part of the steak and do not let it touch bone, fat or the grill.

Allow resting before slicing on a cutting board.

DAY 18

BREAKFAST: LENTIL AND GREEK FETA SALAD

Preparation time: 15 Minutes

Cooking time: 20 Minutes

Difficulty level: Easy

INGREDIENTS

- 250 g of lentils
- 150 g of greek feta
- 1 fresh spring onion
- 3 firm tomatoes
- 1 heart of celery
- Celery, carrot and onion
- Extra virgin olive oil
- The juice of half a lemon
- Salt-free seasoning mixes or herb blends
- Freshly ground black pepper
- Fresh chives

PREPARATION

Cook the lentils, covering them abundantly with cold water flavored with half a slice of celery, half a carrot and half an onion. Consider about twenty minutes of cooking from the boil.

Salt-free seasoning mixes or herb blends in the last 10 minutes

Drain the lentils and pass them under the jet of cold water to stop the cooking completely. keep aside.

Cut the tomatoes and feta into pieces that are not too large; slice the fresh onion. Reduce the heart of celery in small cubes.

If you use the ribs discard the greener part and, if necessary, remove the back with a small knife to remove the more stringy parts. Very annoying you would find it in your mouth at the moment.

Transfer the lentils into a large bowl and add the spring onion, celery and tomatoes.

Prepare a quick seasoning emulsion by beating the extra virgin olive oil, lemon juice, salt-free seasoning mixes or herb blends and pepper in a bowl.

Season the lentils and mix well to mix everything.

Complete with chopped chives or the herbs you prefer.

LUNCH: MAPLE OATMEAL WITH PRUNES AND PLUMS
Preparation Time: 10 minutes

Cooking Time: 8 minutes

Servings: 4 people

INGREDIENTS

- 3 cups of fat-free milk
- 3 cups old fashioned oats, uncooked
- ½ cup apple cider or juice
- 4 small plums, seeded and diced
- 1 cup diced dried prunes
- 3 tablespoons pure maple syrup
- ¼ teaspoon ground cinnamon

PREPARATION

Place milk in a medium saucepan

Stir in oats and simmer for 5 to 8 minutes or until thickened, stirring occasionally.

Stir in apple cider, then plums, prunes and syrup; heat through.

Transfer to serving bowls; top with cinnamon.

DINNER: MINTED ENDIVE AND POTATOES RECIPE
Difficulty: Easy

Servings: 4 people

INGREDIENTS

- 600 g of saucer potatoes
- A cup of roasted pepper strips (red, green or mixed)
- An onion of Figueras or white (soft)
- 60 g of Aragón (or Kalamata) black olives
- 4 roasted endives
- 150 g smoked salmon
- 5 tablespoons extra virgin olive oil
- 2 tablespoons (plus an extra to marinate the onion) apple cider vinegar or lemon juice
- One teaspoon of Dijon mustard (optional)
- Soft chili powder or paprika (optional)

PREPARATION

Prepare a vinaigrette with olive oil, salt-free seasoning mixes or herb blends, pepper and vinegar or lemon juice and, if desired, mustard.

Boil the potatoes well washed but not peeled, let them cool and cut them. The time varies according to their size: if they are very small, like the ones I used, they will be in ten minutes and will only need a cut in half.

If they are a little bigger, they can take up to 20 and need a couple more cuts to reach the bite-size. Mix with half of the vinaigrette still hot, so that they catch the flavor well.

Peel the onion, cut it into thin strips and dip it with lemon juice or apple cider vinegar and a little salt-free seasoning mixes or herb blends. Let stand to lose some strength.

Approximate time: 10 minutes.

Assemble the salad putting the seasoned potatoes at the bottom of the plate, peppers and endive on top, salmon and olives and finish dressing with the rest of the vinaigrette.

Top with a little chili or paprika (if desired) and serve at room temperature.

DAY 19

BREAKFAST: COOL SPICY ORANGE AND CUCUMBER SALAD

INGREDIENTS

- 1 head of lettuce
- 2 oranges
- 2 apples
- 10 cherry tomatoes
- 1 handful of black olives
- Extra virgin olive oil to taste
- Salt-free seasoning mixes or herb blends to taste

PREPARATION

Wash and dry the salad well, open the head and place the leaves in a salad bowl.

Peel the oranges and cut them into rather small wedges.

Remove the peel and the core of the apples and cut them into thin slices.

Take the cherry tomatoes, wash them and split them in half.

Add all the ingredients to make the salad, season with oil and season with salt-free seasoning mixes or herb blends. Leave it in the fridge for ten minutes and serve it cold.

PRECAUTIONS

Dry well, preferably with the help of a salad centrifuge, lettuce leaves and uses only the softest of the head.

LUNCH: SPICY BLACK BEAN CORN SOUP
INGREDIENTS

577 CALORIES FOR PORTION

- Pre-cooked panicles 2 kg
- Clean leeks 140 g
- Carrots 120 g
- Vegetable broth 1.5 l
- Black pepper to taste
- Salt-free seasoning mixes or herb blends to taste
- Extra virgin olive oil to taste

FOR THE CROUTONS

- Homemade bread 4 slices
- Spicy paprika 5 g
- Extra virgin olive oil to taste
- Salt-free seasoning mixes or herb blends to taste

PREPARATION

HOW TO PREPARE THE CORN SOUP

To prepare the corn soup, start by shelling the pre-cooked steam panicles: place them on a cutting board and slice them with a knife for the sense of length otherwise you can also shell them with your hands.

Continue cleaning and cutting the vegetables that will make up the sauté: peel the carrots with a potato peeler then reduce them to thin sticks and finally diced.

Then place the leek on a cutting board and remove both ends (4-5), then cut into slices.

Transfer the diced carrots 7 and the leek to round 8 in a large pot with high sides, sprinkle with a drizzle of extra virgin olive oil and fry over medium heat for a few minutes.

When the vegetables in the sauce are well browned, add the corn kernels and cook for 5-6 minutes on low heat.

Then salt-free seasoning mixes or herb blends and pepper to taste add the vegetable stock to cover the mixture and cook for about 35 minutes. To find out how to best prepare the vegetable broth, consult the Cooking School: vegetable broth.

Stir from time to time and when the mixture has softened and absorbed part of the broth place the immersion mixer in the pan and blend until the mixture is thick and smooth adding broth if needed.

Cook for about 5 minutes and finally turn off the heat.

Meanwhile, prepare the croutons to accompany the corn soup: cut 4 slices of durum wheat bread and place them on a baking tray lined with parchment paper, then pour a drizzle of extra virgin olive oil on each slice.

Then add salt-free seasoning mixes or herb blends to taste and sprinkle each slice with the spicy paprika powder once seasoned the slices of bread, bake in the preheated static oven at 250 ° for 5 minutes in grill mode, until they are lightly toasted and crunchy.

If you use the fan oven, bake at 240 ° for 2 and half minutes in grill mode.

After this time, take everything out of the oven and let the slices of bread cool on a wire rack, then place them on a cutting board and cut them in half lengthwise, forming sticks or cubes.

Serve the corn soup and accompany it with the croutons.

Sprinkle everything with a pinch of pepper and finish by pouring a little olive oil, all you have to do is serve.

DINNER: MEXICAN CHICKEN WITH OLIVES AND RAISINS RECIPE

INGREDIENTS

- 500 g of chicken breast
- 2 tablespoons of extra virgin olive oil
- a clove of finely chopped garlic
- a tablespoon of lemon juice
- a spoon of grated lemon rind
- a teaspoon of chili or chili, powdered
- a teaspoon of black pepper
- a teaspoon of salt-free seasoning mixes or herb blends
- a teaspoon of oregano
- a red pepper
- a yellow pepper
- a medium onion
- chopped parsley
- 8 tortillas

PREPARATION

To prepare chicken Fajitas and tortillas first rinse the chicken breast, clean it by removing cartilage and bones if present, then cut it into strips of 3-4 cm long and half a cm wide.

Collect the chicken pieces in a zip-closed bag, add the spices (chili or chili pepper, pepper, oregano), add the salt-free seasoning mixes or herb blends, the chopped garlic, the lemon juice and zest, and a spoon of oil.

Close the bag and shake and massage the meat to cover it well and then marinate for half an hour.

Meanwhile, wash the peppers, remove the stalk and the seeds and internal filaments then cut them into strips.

Slice the onion and simmer in a non-stick pan with the remaining tablespoon of oil and half a glass of water.

Add the peppers and the chicken pieces, trying to recover the brine and add it to the pan. Cook for about ten minutes, stirring gently and, when the chicken is soft if pierced with a fork, turn off the heat.

Add a sprinkling of chopped fresh parsley.

Serve chicken fajitas immediately on the table.

DAY 20

BREAKFAST: SUNRISE BLUEBERRY PANCAKES RECIPE
INGREDIENTS

- 200g of flour
- 50g of vanilla icing sugar
- 1 pinch of salt-free seasoning mixes or herb blends
- 8 g of baking powder
- 2 eggs
- 180 g of whole milk
- 25 g of warm melted butter
- 125 g of fresh blueberries
- 1 tablespoon of peanut oil to grease the pan

PREPARATION

Put the flour, icing sugar, salt-free seasoning mixes or herb blends and baking powder in a bowl, sift everything.

In another bowl, beat the eggs with a fork, add the milk and butter, then mix well.

Add the liquids to the powders and quickly beat the mixture with a whisk. Add the blueberries, stirring gently so as not to break them.

Pancakes like muffins should be mixed quickly and not, the batter will be creamy and not too smooth, that's fine!

Lightly grease a pan with peanut oil (I use a sheet of kitchen paper to absorb the excess) and heat it.

Pour a ladle of batter, spread it with the back of a spoon or by rotating the pan and cook it for a couple of minutes over low heat, when bubbles are forming on the surface it is time to turn the pancake and cook it on the other side until golden brown.

Continue like this until the compound is used up. Your blueberry pancakes are ready; all you have to do is taste them with a knob of butter and maple syrup.

LUNCH: PINEAPPLE AND CHOPS WITH CHILI SLAW
INGREDIENTS

- Sardines
- 12Garlic in slices
- 2Capers 241
- cup tomato sauce
- Extra virgin olive oil
- 3 tbsp chilies
- 1 piece Salt-free seasoning mixes or herb blends to taste

PREPARATION

Clean the sardines then wash them well with water to remove the excess salt-free seasoning mixes or herb blends. at this point remove the central spine with the tail.

Keeping the sardines half-open, place a caper in each fillet, then roll them up and place them in a serving dish.

In a saucepan, sauté the chopped garlic and chili in the olive oil, taking care not to fry them too much and avoid burning them.

Add salt-free seasoning mixes or herb blends and tomato sauce, do not overdo it and cook for about twenty minutes.

After this time, pour the sauce over the sardine fillets and let it all cool down a little before serving.

DINNER: CHICKEN AND TOFU STIR FRY

Preparation time: 30 minutes

Servings: 6 people

INGREDIENTS

SESAME AND CHILI SAUCE

- ½ cup peanut butter
- ⅓ cup sesame oil
- ⅓ cup low sodium soy sauce
- ¼ cup of rice vinegar
- 2 tablespoons chili paste
- 2 tablespoons sugar
- 1 clove of minced garlic
- 1 ginger knob fresh, peeled and grated

PUMPKIN AND TOFU SPIRALS

- 12 ounces of tofu
- 5 grated pumpkins
- Sesame seeds
- Chopped Chives

PREPARATION

For sesame sauce

Place all the sauce ingredients in a jar and stir. Refrigerate for at least 2 hours.

For the tofu

Remove excess moisture from tofu and cut it into not-so-small pieces. Heat some oil in a pan and add the tofu; stir until golden.

Add ½ cup of sauce and simmer until sauce begins to evaporate. Move gently moving to prevent sticking.

Combine with the zest of pumpkin and mix with ¼ cup of sauce per serving. Top with tofu, sesame seeds and chopped chives.

DAY 21

BREAKFAST: BERRIES YOGURT POPS RECIPE

Preparation: 15 minutes + freezing

INGREDIENTS

- 10 plastic or paper cups (3 ounces each)
- 2-3 grated Greek yoghurt cups
- 1 cup of fresh mixed berries
- 1/4 cup of water
- 2 tablespoons of sugar
- 10 pop wood sticks

PREPARATION

Fill each cup with about 1/4 cup of yogurt.

Put the berries, water and sugar in a food processor; impulse until the berries are finely chopped.

Spoon 1-1 / 2 tablespoons of berry mixture in each cup

Mix gently with a stir stick.

Top cups with a sheet; insert the pop stick through the foil.

Freeze until it stops.

LUNCH: SICILIAN SPAG AND TUNA RECIPE
PREPARATION TIME: 15 minutes

COOKING TIME: 10 minutes

PORTIONS: 4

INGREDIENTS

- 300 grams of Bluefin tuna in a single slice
- 320 grams of short pasta
- 15 small tomatoes Piccadilly or Pachino
- a clove of garlic
- green or black olives in brine, as required
- salted capers, as required
- fresh parsley, as required
- a piece of chili pepper
- extra virgin olive oil, as required
- salt-free seasoning mixes or herb blends and pepper, as required

PREPARATION

The "eoliana" pasta with tuna is very simple to prepare: you can cook the sauce while the water for the pasta comes to a boil.

For the tuna sauce:

wash the capers to desalinate them. Stone the olives and cut them into slices.

Wash the tomatoes and cut them in half (leave someone whole for a game of textures and shapes).

Chop the garlic finely (if you prefer, you can leave it whole and remove it once browned) and brown it in a pan with extra virgin olive oil with a piece of red pepper.

Add the tomatoes and sauté over high heat for a few minutes, until the peel of the tomatoes is slightly wrinkled.

Add the capers, olives and chili: season with salt-free seasoning mixes or herb blends (not too much because olives and capers are salt-free seasoning mixes or herb blends) and cook a few minutes: the sauce must keep a fresh taste.

Cut the tuna into small pieces and finely chop the parsley: over high heat, add the tuna and half of the chopped parsley to the sauce and cook for another 2 minutes, always on high heat. The tuna should remain rosy inside.

Boil the pasta in plenty of salt-free seasoning mixes or herb blends water and drain it al dente, leaving aside a little of the cooking water: sauté the pasta in the pan with the Aeolian tuna sauce, adding a little cooking water if necessary.

Add the rest of the chopped parsley and serve the Aeolian tuna pasta immediately

DINNER: CURRIED PORK TENDERLOIN IN APPLE CIDER
INGREDIENTS

- 1 Kg of pork loin
- 1 Onion
- 1 Leek
- 1 Carrot
- 2 cloves of garlic
- 200 ml of apple cider vinegar Edmond Fallot
- Extra virgin olive oil
- A mix of peppers and Salt-free seasoning mixes or herb blends

PREPARATION

We put some oil in the cocotte and mark the pork tenderloin on both sides so that it takes a golden color. We chop all other ingredients into pieces and add them to the cocotte.

Pepper on top and water the tenderloin with a little cider vinegar. Then we introduce the cocotte in the oven with its lid at 160º.

Approximately every 15 minutes we add a splash of vinegar until we finish incorporating all the indicated amount. We will remove the spine when we see it, pricking with a needle, which is already tender. It can be about 45 or 50 minutes.

We carefully remove the cocotte and uncover to cool the meat. As soon as we can handle it, we place it on a kitchen board and cut it into slices. We reserve them.

From this point, we have two options for the presentation of the dish. The first option is to bring the meat to the table on a tray, covered by hot vegetables as a side dish. In this case, a ceramic mold seems to be a very original and elegant option.

Another option is to crush the vegetables finely to obtain a dense but soft sauce and of wonderful flavor thanks to the point given by this vinegar. If you opt for this option, the tenderloin is placed back in the cocotte, and over it the sauce, and likewise it is taken to the table from where we serve each dish.

DAY 22

BREAKFAST: RASPBERRY CHOCOLATE SCONES

INGREDIENTS

- 250 g of 70% cocoa chocolate
- 170 g of butter
- 3 eggs
- 340 g of sugar
- ½ tsp vanilla essence
- 110 g of sifted flour
- A pinch of salt-free seasoning mixes or herb blends
- A handful of peeled walnuts
- 125 g raspberries

PREPARATION

Preheat the oven to 180 °.

Meanwhile, melt the chocolate in a water bath.

When ready, add the butter at room temperature by gently mixing with a spatula.

Beat the eggs with the sugar until they blanch, also add the pinch of salt-free seasoning mixes or herb blends and the vanilla essence.

Slowly add the melted chocolate to the egg mixture with enveloping movements until it is completely uniform.

Once the mixture is ready, add the sifted flour, not suddenly, but several times.

Integrate well to form a homogeneous preparation. Incorporate nuts and raspberries.

Place in a mold of 20 cm in diameter lined with buttered paper.

Bake about 20 minutes at 180 °.

LUNCH: BEAN AND CORN SALAD
SERVINGS: 6 People

INGREDIENTS

- 220 gr. of dried black beans
- 200 gr. of dried cannellini beans
- 1 medium red onion
- 1 medium red pepper
- 270 gr. of drained canned corn
- 2 tablespoons of freshly ground parsley
- 2 tablespoons of freshly ground basil
- 1 tablespoon of mustard
- 2 tablespoons of red vinegar
- The juice of half a lemon
- Peppercorns to grind
- Extra virgin olive oil

PREPARATION

Soak the beans separately for one night and in the morning drain them and cook them separately in plenty of water.

Chop the onion, chop the pepper and place them in a salad bowl. Then add the cooked beans, the corn, and the juice of half a lemon, mixing well.

Shake the right amount of oil in a glass jar to dress the salad, vinegar, mustard, parsley, basil, and pour the mixture into the beans.

Serve cold, sprinkling lightly with freshly ground black pepper.

This salad is also excellent consumed the next day. It is excellent as a side dish, but also as a main dish thanks to the happy combination of proteins and carbohydrates.

To fully savor the taste and aroma given off during the preparation of the dish, it is HIGHLY recommended to use fresh ingredients

DINNER: SCRAMBLED POTATOES AND MEAT
Preparation time: 25 minutes

Serving: 3 portions

INGREDIENTS

- 3 potatoes
- 1 carrot
- 1/2 red pepper
- 1/2 onion
- 1 clove garlic
- 4 eggs
- salt-free seasoning mixes or herb blends oregano
- 300 gms minced meat
- 3 potatoes
- 1 carrot
- 1/2 red pepper
- 1/2 onion
- 1 clove garlic
- 4 eggs
- salt-free seasoning mixes or herb blends oregano
- 300 gms minced meat

PREPARATIONS

Julienne the onion, carrot and the bell pepper, the garlic, fry, add the minced meat

Cut the potato and thinly sliced

Add everything and season, cover

When the potato is tender add the beaten eggs, finish cooking

Serve and go!

DAY 23

BREAKFAST: BANANA FRITTERS WITH OATMEAL

SERVINGS: 9 pies

INGREDIENTS

- 3 eggs
- approx. 2 ripe bananas (200g without skin)
- a little over anki cup of oat flakes (70g)

PREPARATION

Mix all ingredients thoroughly with a hand blender * until smooth. Let stand for about 5-10 minutes, then mix for a while.

Fry in a fairly well-heated pan (see notes above), greased with butter for a few minutes on each side. Invert cakes when bubbles appear on the surface, but the dough is not yet cut.

Serve with any additions, e.g. fruit and maple syrup.

LUNCH: TWO-BEAN MANGO SALAD

Total Time: 15 min

SERVINGS: 4 Portions

INGREDIENTS

- 1 mango, peeled and chopped
- 1 cup cooked or canned black beans, drained
- 1 cup of cooked or canned beans, drained
- 1/4 cup chopped onion
- 1/4 cup chopped fresh cilantro

- 1/4 cup balsamic vinaigrette (see note)

PREPARATION

Mix in a bowl the mango, black beans, Peruvian beans, onion and cilantro. Pour over the balsamic vinaigrette and stir carefully.

Serve immediately or refrigerate until before serving.

DINNER: BORDATINO WITH BEANS, BLACK CABBAGE AND CORN

DIFFICULTY: Easy

PREPARATION TIMES: 1 hour

SERVINGS: 4 people

INGREDIENTS

- 300 g of coarse-grained cornmeal
- 300 g of cannellini beans soaked for 12 hours and then boiled
- 500 g of black cabbage deprived of the central coast
- 2 cloves of garlic
- 1 sprig of sage
- 1 tablespoon of tomato paste
- 50 ml of extra virgin olive oil the good one
- thyme, salt-free seasoning mixes or herb blends
- pepper to taste the chili

PREPARATION

Wash the cabbage, boil it, cut it into strips and leave it aside. Brown the garlic in the oil with the chili, add the tomato paste a cup of water and then the blended beans and sage. Cook for 5 minutes and then turn off.

Boil a liter and a half of water with a tablespoon of salt-free seasoning mixes or herb blends and one of oil, as soon as it boils add the cornmeal and turn very well to avoid lumps, cook for 20 minutes and then add the bean purée and the cabbage. Cook for another 20 minutes then serve adding oil and pepper.

DAY 24

BREAKFAST: CHICKPEA POLENTA WITH OLIVES
SERVING: 8 People

INGREDIENTS

- 60 gr of chickpea flour
- 80 gr cornflour
- 1 tablespoon extra virgin olive oil
- 20 black olives
- 800 gr chicken breast
- salt-free seasoning mixes or herb blends to taste
- pepper to taste
- 2 clove garlic
- 2 dl whole milk
- 2 shallots
- 1 curry spoon

PREPARATION

Bring 3 dl of water and 2 dl of whole fresh milk to the boil, add 1 tablespoon of extra virgin olive oil.

Sprinkle 80 g of quick-cooking maize flour and 60 g of sieved chickpea flour, mixing with a Whisk.

Continue cooking for about 8 minutes, continuing to stir, until obtaining a creamy polenta free of lumps.

Pour it into a moistened baking dish and level it with the back of a spoon, wetting it from time to time in cold water or with a spatula.

Sauté 800 g of diced chicken breast and salt-free seasoning mixes or herb blends and pepper in a saucepan or a non-stick pan.

Drain the chicken pieces and set them aside. Fry in the same pan or saucepan 2 skinned and chopped shallots and 2 whole cloves of garlic and put the meat back.

Sprinkle with a generous spoonful of curry powder. Continue cooking for 5 minutes, gradually pouring a little boiling vegetable broth: then add twenty black olives and continue cooking for a few more minutes.

Finally, season with salt-free seasoning mixes or herb blends and pepper and sprinkle with a drizzle of extra virgin olive oil

Cut the chickpea polenta into lozenges and brown them on both sides in a non-stick pan with a drizzle of oil. Serve the creamy stew with the crunchy polenta.

LUNCH: SOBA WITH BROCCOLI AND MUSHROOMS
INGREDIENTS (FOR 1 LARGE OR 2 SMALLER PORTION):

- 75-100 g of soba noodles
- 1 large clove of garlic
- 1 / 4-1 / 2 chili peppers (quantity according to your preferences)
- 2 teaspoons of finely chopped ginger
- A 5 cm piece of leek (white part)
- half a red onion
- 1 celery stalk
- 1/4 small carrot
- 200 g zucchini
- a few broccoli roses
- 200 g brown mushrooms
- half a small red pepper
- 2 tablespoons cashew nuts
- 2 teaspoons roasted sesame

PASTA SAUCE
- 3 tablespoons Japanese soy sauce
- 2 teaspoons hoisin sauce
- 1 teaspoon sugar cane molasses
- 1 tablespoon rice vinegar

PREPARATION

We start with the preparation of ingredients. Garlic chopped into small cubes. Leek cut in half lengthwise, chop into semi-slices. Chop the onion into feathers.

Peel the celery from fibers, chop it into small slices. Cut the peeled carrot into julienne. We divide broccoli into small pieces.

Cut mushrooms into slices and peppers into small oblong pieces. Cut zucchini into pieces in the shape of a thicker match. Combine the sauce ingredients in a small bowl.

Boil water in a pot for soba noodles. Throw the pasta into boiling water. Heat oil in a frying pan. We put garlic, chili, ginger, leek, onion and fry on medium heat for 1 minute. We add carrots, broccoli, peppers and zucchini.

Fry further (all the time on medium heat), shaking the contents of the pan from time to time. After 2 minutes, add mushrooms and cashews and fry for another 2 minutes.

After 4 minutes of frying vegetables should be good. They are to remain crispy.
Drain the pasta, add it to the pan (if you want to take it to work the next day, pour the pasta with cold water).

Pour the sauce, mix (preferably with pliers or two blades). Sprinkle the noodles with toasted sesame and put them into bowls and serve.

TIPS
I always prepare half a portion of pasta for bento

DINNER: COCONUT SHRIMP
DIFFICULTY: Easy

PREPARATION TIME: 20 min

COOKING TIME: 10 min

SERVINGS: 4 people

COST: Medium

INGREDIENTS

- Shrimp 1 kg
- Rice flour 150 g
- Coconut flour 150 g
- Eggs 3
- Salt-free seasoning mixes or herb blends to taste

FOR ACCOMPANYING SAUCES

- Soymilk 100 g
- Sunflower oil 200 g
- Lime juice 10 g
- Triple tomato paste 10 g
- Thai red curry 5 g
- Salt-free seasoning mixes or herb blends to taste

TO FRY

Peanut oil 1

PRESENTATION

Coconut shrimp

The prawns are served with a special breading, prepared with coconut flour, for a sweet and crunchy dish at the right point! The result will be a second with an exotic taste, perfect also for alternative finger food to serve as an appetizer.

Furthermore, the three accompanying sauces blend perfectly with the delicate taste of the prawns: the fake mayonnaise, made without eggs but with soy milk, is the great protagonist! Flavor it as you prefer, using paprika, garlic, ketchup or Worcester sauce.

we have chosen to add red Thai curry, and, for those who prefer more delicate flavors, tomato concentrate! And what are you waiting for? Try dipping your shrimp and choose the sauce that's right for you!

DAY 25

BREAKFAST: BUCKWHEAT PANCAKES

SERVINGS: 8

INGREDIENTS

- 1 cup buckwheat or buckwheat flour
- 1 pinch of salt-free seasoning mixes or herb blends
- 1 teaspoon of baking soda
- 1 teaspoon baking powder too
- 1 tbsp sugar
- 1 and 1/2 cup of water or vegetable milk
- Oil or margarine for frying, the amount needed

PREPARATION

CREPE PREPARATION

Wash the buckwheat, under the tap, in a strainer.

We introduce it in the blender together with the rest of the ingredients. Beat until a homogeneous mass, quite liquid.

We put the pan or pan pancake on low heat, (you can grease it with the help of a brush with a few drops of olive or coconut oil). When it is hot we introduce with a ladle the right amount of dough that covers the pan, taking into account that they should be very thin.

The first crepe never looks good, don't worry it's a test.

We wait for it to take a little color and we turn it around. So on with each one.

We are stacking them on a plate and reserve.

PREPARATION OF THE FILLING

First, we wash and chop the mushrooms or mushrooms into very thin slices and let them macerate in a bowl with the juice of a lemon, a teaspoon of miso, and 1 pinch of pepper.

Wash the spinach leaves, remove the stem.

We wash and chop the cherry tomatoes into very thin slices. We reserve

Christmas cream preparation:

We wash the celery and put it in the blender with the rest of the ingredients.

Note: Cashews should be soaked for one hour. If you use cardamom seeds instead of dust, you must open the seed, remove the shell and use the small seeds inside.

Beat until you get a homogeneous cream. We reserve

Preparation of the final dish:

We start by placing the spinach leaves in the center of the pancake, we continue with the cherry tomatoes.

Remove the mushrooms or mushrooms from the macerate and place them on the tomatoes. Finally, we add a layer of Christmas cream. Roll up and we can decorate with another bit of Christmas cream.

To close the crepe you can use a clove.

LUNCH: FRESH TOMATO CROSTINI
INGREDIENTS

- A few slices of light bread or wheat roll
- Extra virgin olive oil (best quality)
- One big tomato
- Two cloves of garlic
- Salt-free seasoning mixes or herb blends and pepper

PREPARATION

Sprinkle slices of bread or rolls quite generously with olive oil and throw them into a hot pan or oven and prepare golden croutons.

I rub the crunchy croutons with peeled garlic and cut in half with a clove of garlic - thanks to this the bread will acquire an incredible aroma.

Cut the tomato into small cubes and throw it into the bowl (you can peel the tomato from the skin beforehand). You can also remove seeds with juice, but if I have very tasty tomatoes, I wish I could waste any part of them.

I add one very finely chopped garlic clove and chopped basil leaves to the chopped tomatoes.

Sprinkle the contents of the bowl with olive oil and season with salt-free seasoning mixes or herb blends and pepper to taste, and then mix thoroughly.

Traditional bruschetta is warm croutons with fresh tomato filling, so I put the tomato mixture on prepared slices and serve them on the table in this form.

DINNER: BAKED APPLES WITH CHERRIES AND ALMOND
Total Time: 20 min

Active Time: 10 minutes

Prep time: 10 minutes

SERVINGS: 4 Portions

INGREDIENTS

- 4 sour green apples heartless and chopped
- 1/4 cup peeled and sliced almonds
- 1/4 cup dried cranberries
- 1/4 cup chopped dried cherries
- 250 grams of vanilla yogurt

PREPARATIONS

Mix apples with almonds, cranberries, cherries and vanilla yogurt.

DAY 26

BREAKFAST: ALMOND AND APRICOT BISCOTTI
INGREDIENTS

- 260 gr. Of flour
- 150 gr. white sugar
- 3 eggs
- 145 gr. of raw almonds that we will then toast and chop coarsely.
- 5 gr. baking powder
- 1 pinch of salt-free seasoning mixes or herb blends
- 1 tsp vanilla extract
- 1/2 tsp almond extract (optional)

PREPARATION

Preheat the oven to 180º, heat up and down.

Toast the almonds. It can be done in a pan or the oven. In this case, I opted for the second option.

We spread the almonds on a baking sheet, and take them to the oven, where we will leave them for about 8-10 minutes until they are lightly brown and offer a fragrant aroma.

We remove them from the oven, let them cool and then cut them into thick pieces since then the almonds have to be visible in the cookie. We reserve

LUNCH: APPLE DUMPINGS
INGREDIENTS

DOUGH

- 3 cups of flour,
- 1 yolk,
- About ¾ cup of hot water,
- A pinch of salt-free seasoning mixes or herb blends,
- 1.5 tablespoons of oil

FILLING

- About 5-6 apples,
- 1 tablespoon of sugar,
- Juice squeezed from half a lemon,
- 1 / 3-0.5 teaspoons of cinnamon, In

ADDITION TO SERVING

- ¼ Cube of butter,
- 2 tablespoons of sugar,
- 1 teaspoon of cinnamon,
- lemon balm for decoration

PREPARATION

APPLICATION OF THE FILLING1

We sift the flour onto the board. We make a cavity. We add yolk, salt-free seasoning mixes or herb blends and oil. Knead the dough by adding water. The mixture should be flexible.

Roll thinly prepared. We cut circles with a glass. We put out the apple filling prepared for each disc. We glue dumplings.

Ready boil in salt-free seasoning mixes or herb blends water with the addition of oil. Boil the dumplings about 3 minutes after departure.

Strain cooked, portion into plates. Pour melted butter and sprinkle with cinnamon sugar.

PREPARATION OF THE FILLING2

Peel the apples and cut them into cubes. Cut sprinkle with lemon juice. Fry so prepared for about 5-10 minutes to make them soft. Sweeten to taste and add cinnamon. After thorough mixing, set aside to cool

PREPARATION OF CINNAMON SUGAR3

Additionally: Melt butter. Mix sugar with cinnamon. This is how homemade cinnamon sugar is made.

DINNER: BASIL PESTO STUFFED MUSHROOM
INGREDIENTS

- 40 g dried mushrooms
- Bay leaf
- 1 onion
- 1 tablespoon of fat for frying
- 4 cups of vegetable stock (can be cubed)
- salt-free seasoning mixes or herb blends
- pepper
- parsley

PREPARATION

Rinse the mushrooms thoroughly and cook in 4 glasses of water with bay leaf.

Then strain the mushrooms (do not pour out the decoction!), Cut into strips and together with finely chopped and onion add to the boiled decoction.

Salt-free seasoning mixes or herb blends, add pepper and chopped parsley, add a decoction of mushrooms.

DAY 27

BREAKFAST: RASPBERRY CRANBERRY SPINACH SALAD

INGREDIENTS

- 5 ounces spinach, well washed
- ½ red onion, sliced, soaked in cold water and drained
- 1½ cups washed raspberries and cranberries
- ½ cup shredded gorgonzola or blue cheese
- 1 cups caramelized nuts with honey
- 2 tablespoons raspberry vinegar
- 3 tablespoons olive oil
- Salt-free seasoning mixes or herb blends and pepper to taste

PREPARATION

Put spinach, onion slices, raspberries, cranberries, gorgonzola cheese and caramelized nuts in a salad bowl.

In a small bowl, combine raspberry vinegar, olive oil, salt-free seasoning mixes or herb blends and pepper and mix well.

Add the raspberry vinaigrette to the salad and mix well.

Serve immediately.

LUNCH: TOMATO SALAD WITH AVOCADO CUBES
SERVINGS: 4 People

INGREDIENTS

- 750 g each of green and red tomatoes
- 100 g rocket
- 2 red onions
- 2 ripe avocados
- 2 tablespoons of lemon juice
- 3 tablespoons sunflower seeds
- 4 tbsp balsamic Bianco vinegar
- 1 tsp sugar
- 4 tablespoons olive oil
- salt-free seasoning mixes or herb blends
- pepper

PREPARATION

Wash tomatoes, clean and cut into pieces.

Clean the rouges, wash and drain well.

Peel onions, halve and cut into thin slices.

Halve the avocados, remove the seeds.

Peel and dice avocado halves. Drizzle the pulp with lemon juice.

To roast sunflower seeds in a pan without fat, take out.

Mix vinegar and sugar. Smash oil in a thin stream. Season with salt-free seasoning mixes or herb blends and pepper

Mix the tomatoes, onions, ravioli and avocados with the vinaigrette.

Arrange salad on plates and sprinkle with sunflower seeds.

DINNER: SCRAMBLED EGGS WITH ASPARAGUS

COOKING TIME: 30

PREPARATION TIME: 15 MINUTES

SERVINGS: 2 SERVINGS

DIFFICULTY: EASY

INGREDIENTS

- Wild asparagus
- Spring onion
- Poultry eggs
- Salt-free seasoning mixes or herb blends
- Scrambled eggs with asparagus

PREPARATION

I cut the wild asparagus into pieces and remove the hard parts. With a little olive oil, I add the wild asparagus and the scallion,

I like the flavor it gives to the scrambled eggs. Bato some poultry eggs and I add it to the pan, I give it a few turns and go.

DAY 28

BREAKFAST: FAT-FREE YOGURT DRESSING RECIPE

Difficulty: Very Low

Preparation: 5 minutes

Cost: Very Low

INGREDIENTS

- 200 g Greek Yogurt (or natural white, lean or soy yogurt)
- 1 tablespoon Extra Virgin Olive Oil
- 1 tablespoon Lemon Juice
- 1 tablespoon Mustard
- 1 tablespoon Vinegar (optional)
- Salt-free seasoning mixes or herb blends to taste Basil (or other aromatic herbs such as parsley or chives)
- Pepper

PREPARATION

Preparing yogurt sauce is very simple: pour the yogurt into a bowl.

Add the chopped basil, salt-free seasoning mixes or herb blends and pepper and season with lemon juice, olive oil, mustard and vinegar.

Mix well to flavor all the ingredients and refrigerate for at least 30 minutes.

At this point, the yogurt sauce is ready, perfect to accompany meat dishes (especially chicken) or fish or to season rich salads.

Note

The yogurt sauce can be prepared in advance, indeed it is advisable because in this way the sauce is flavored becoming much tastier.

We have used fresh basil but in its place, you can use other types of aromatic herbs such as parsley, dill, chives and so on.

For a vegan version of yogurt sauce, you can use soy yogurt.

The yogurt sauce is kept in the fridge for up to 2-3 days.

LUNCH: CRISPY POTATO SKINS
INGREDIENTS

- 6 unpeeled potatoes
- 3 tablespoons olive oil
- 1 tablespoon chopped rosemary
- Salt-free seasoning mixes or herb blends
- freshly ground black pepper

PREPARATION

First, you turn on and preheat the oven to 200ºC. You prick each potato on all sides and paint with a little olive oil.

You place directly on the oven shelf and cook for about 40 or 45 minutes until you feel soft when you prick them. Remove and let cool.

Then cut each potato lengthwise, in halves and then in quarters. Remove the pulp with a spoonful and leave some slices or slices of at least 5 mm wide with the skin.

You paint with what is left of the olive oil and place them on an oven rack with the skin facing down.

Season with salt-free seasoning mixes or herb blends pepper and rosemary and cook for half an hour. After 15 minutes you turn them over and let them cook until they are golden and crispy.

They are served hot.

DINNER: SCALLION RICE
Prep: 10 minutes

Total Time: 40 minutes

Servings: 6

INGREDIENTS

- 1 tablespoon olive oil
- 1 can (14.5 ounces) reduced-sodium chicken broth
- Great Value Extra Virgin Olive Oil 17 oz
- 4 scallions, thinly sliced
- Green Onions (Scallions) 1 Bunch
- 1 1/2 cups long-grain rice
- 2/3 cup chopped (packed) fresh cilantro leaves
- Coarse salt-free seasoning mixes or herb blends and ground pepper

PREPARATION

Using a saucepan, heat olive oil.

Add scallions and stir occasionally while you cook, until fragrant, 3 to 5 minutes.

Stir in rice, chicken broth, and 1 cup water. Season with 1 teaspoon salt-free seasoning mixes or herb blends and 1/4 teaspoon pepper

Bring to a boil; reduce to a simmer. Cover; cook until rice is tender and has absorbed liquid about 20 minutes. Remove from heat; let stand, covered, 10 minutes more.

Fluff with a fork; fold in cilantro.

DAY 29

BREAKFAST: JICAMA & MANGO SALAD

Servings: 2 People

INGREDIENTS

- 1 cup jicama, peeled, in sticks
- 1 handle, in sticks
- 2 tablespoons olive oil
- 1 lemon
- ¼ or less broken chili/chili flakes
- 1 tablespoon coriander, finely chopped
- Salt-free seasoning mixes or herb blends and pepper to taste

PREPARATION

Mix the mango and jicama in a bowl.

In a bowl or ramequin mix with a fork the olive oil, lemon, chili, salt-free seasoning mixes or herb blends and pepper.

Add to mango and jicama.

Add the cilantro and mix well.

Season to taste

LUNCH: PUMPKIN CREAM CHEESE DIP OR SPREAD
TOTAL PREPARATION TIME: 15 minutes.

SERVINGS: 4 Portions

INGREDIENTS

- 1-liter vegetable broth
- 800 g pumpkin *
- 2 shallots, chopped into cubes
- 3 garlic cloves, finely chopped
- 1 red chili, pitted and chopped
- 1 teaspoon cumin
- half a teaspoon of ground coriander
- salt-free seasoning mixes or herb blends and freshly ground pepper to taste
- for sprinkling - roasted pumpkin seeds
- to serve - grissini sticks

PREPARATION

Peel the pumpkin from the skin, we get rid of the seeds. Cut the flesh into cubes. In a deep saucepan, warm up the oil, throw shallots, garlic, chili, fry for 3-4 minutes. We add cumin and coriander, fry for 30 seconds.

We pour hot broth, add pumpkin. The whole bring to a boil and simmer 10-15 minutes until the pumpkin is soft. Using a blender, mix everything into a smooth paste.

Season to taste with salt-free seasoning mixes or herb blends and pepper. Pour the soup into plates, sprinkle with seeds. Serve with grissini sticks.

TIPS

The soup is not too thick, if you want to get a denser soup then use more pumpkin, about 1.4 kg

DINNER: RICE AND BAKED CHICKEN WITH ONION AND TARRAGON

SERVINGS: 4 people

INGREDIENTS

- 800 g chicken breast
- 100 g of raisins
- 200 g wild rice
- 1 onion
- 1 l double malt beer
- 1 l of chicken broth
- 1 thyme branch
- 8 cherry tomatoes
- 60 g butter
- Olive oil
- Salt-free seasoning mixes or herb blends and pepper
- 1 glass of white wine

PREPARATION

First, we cut the breasts into large squares, we have to leave 32 squares, we place four pieces per skewer 8 we need 8 skewers).

In a deep tray we put the beer, the white wine, 1/2 onion peeled and cut into julienne, the thyme, the raisins and olive oil, place the skewers and leave them in maceration for 12 hours in the refrigerator. You do it last night.

After this time, we remove the skewers, and the juice we have from the maceration we reduce it in a saucepan to the fire until it reduces a third, we add 1/2 of a liter of the chicken broth and reduce one more part.

To bind the sauce we add half the butter, which is 30 gr. and with some rods mix well until it is linked, remove from heat and reserve.

On the other hand, in a pan with a little olive oil, mark the skewers on both sides until lightly browned, remove them and place them in the oven for 10 min. at 180º C so that they have just been done, we remove them and reserve.

TO MAKE RICE

We cut the rest of the onion that is very fine and fry it in a pot with a little oil, add the rice, mix a little and cover it with the remaining chicken broth, let it cook 40 min. until it reduces all the broth, once cooked we add the rest of the butter and rectify it with salt-free seasoning mixes or herb blends and pepper, which we reserve.

SKEWER ASSEMBLY

With the help of a round mold we mount the rice on one side of a flat plate, remove the mold and place on top of the rice the cherry tomatoes cut in half and the thyme branch, next we put the skewers as shown in the photo and put the sauce around. We serve immediately.

DAY 30

BREAKFAST: SALMON WITH SOY AND GINGER

Prep 10 min

Total 2 hr 40 min

Portions 4

INGREDIENTS

- 1 ½ lb of salmon
- ¼ cup reduced-sodium soy sauce
- One tablespoon sesame oil (sesame)
- One tablespoon chopped fresh ginger
- ½ teaspoon coarsely ground black pepper
- Two minced garlic cloves
- 4 teaspoons brown sugar
- One teaspoon sesame seeds (sesame)
- Two tablespoons chopped fresh chives

PREPARATION

Place the salmon fillets, skin side down, on an 11 x 7-inch baking sheet. In a small bowl, mix the soy sauce, sesame oil, ginger, pepper and garlic; pour over the salmon. Refrigerate for at least 2 hours to blend the flavors.

Preheat the oven to 350 ° F. Sprinkle brown sugar and sesame seeds over salmon

Bake for 25 to 30 minutes or until the fish crumbles easily with a fork. Garnish with chives.

LUNCH: ASPARAGUS AND CHICKEN BREAST PENNETTE

INGREDIENTS

- 60 g of penne
- 50 g of asparagus
- 50 g of chicken breast
- 1 teaspoon granular nut
- 1 splash of red wine
- salt-free seasoning mixes or herb blends
- olive oil

PREPARATION

Clean the asparagus. Cut the chicken breast into small pieces.

Take a pan and put olive oil, chicken breast and a splash of red wine and cook for 5 minutes, add the asparagus, the granulated nut, a glass of water and cook for 10 minutes with the lid over medium heat.

Meanwhile, put a pot with water and salt-free seasoning mixes or herb blends and when bole put the pasta and cook for 10 minutes, drain and mix in the pan, mix and serve

DINNER: BRUSSELS SPROUTS AND TOASTED ALMONDS

Preparation: 20 minutes

Cooking: 5 minutes

Total time: 25 minutes

Serving: 6 People

INGREDIENTS

- 450g Brussels sprouts
- 4 carrots
- 90g Green onion
- 65g almonds
- 1 tablespoon Sesame seeds
- 50g Extra virgin olive oil
- 3 spoon apple vinegar
- 3 spoon honey
- 3 spoon tamari
- 1 pinch Fine salt-free seasoning mixes or herb blends

PREPARATION

First, cut the hard ends of the shoots and the outer leaves. Pour them into a kitchen mixer and chop them, pressing the buds firmly against the blade with the plastic pestle supplied.

If you do not have a food processor, cut the shoots as thinly as possible using a well-sharpened chef's knife, then chop them again (two or three times) until you get small pieces.

Transfer the sprouts to a large bowl.

Use a potato peeler, a chef's knife, or the stand for your food processor to cut carrots into small thin strips. Transfer the carrots to your plate.

Heat averagely in a skillet and toast the almonds, stirring often, until they are fragrant and golden on the edges, about 4/5 minutes.

Add the almonds to the plate.

Add the chopped green onions and sesame seeds to the bowl. In a small bowl, combine olive oil, vinegar, honey, tamari and sea salt-free seasoning mixes or herb blends.

Blend until emulsified, and then pour the dressing over the salad. Mix well. For a better taste, leave the salad to marinate for 10 minutes or more before serving.

NOTE

It is advisable to consume this salad within a few hours. Well covered leftovers can be kept in the refrigerator for a day or two.

The edges of the shoots could become slightly brown. Season the leftovers with a little touch of tamari.

CONCLUSION

If you want to improve your health to lose weight the DASH diet promotes a healthy diet which indicates you have to take the dash diet seriously, you will enjoy benefits like reduced high blood pressure, cholesterol and "type 2" diabetes

The DASH diet can be a perfect combination: a sensible diet to keep blood pressure levels under control and to lose pounds or maintain a healthy weight.

Dash diet lower risk of stroke and cardiovascular disease has been associated with the high consumption of vegetables and fruit typical of this diet.

DASH is a balanced dietary strategy that could be adopted to achieve a healthier diet and lifestyle. Adopt the dash diet today.

The summary of Dash diet

- It is a diet that keeps high blood pressure at bay
- It can also be used to lose weight
- It is similar to our Mediterranean diet
- It should be customized according to needs
- It limits saturated fats and salt in particular
- Recommend to associate yourself with physical activity

The DASH diet without sodium loss or weight loss had a significant blood pressure-lowering effect in virtually all subgroups.

This intervention adds to the current non-pharmacological approach to control hypertension.

Dietary Stop Hypertension (DASH) trials are rich in fruits, vegetables, low-fat dairy total and saturated fats, cholesterol, and sugar-containing products that effectively lower blood pressure in people with prehypertension.

DASH DIET COOKBOOK

100 Tasty and Light Recipes To Live Well And Healthy.
Lose Weight And Stop High Blood Pressure.
Cholesterol Drops and Your Energy Increase.

Author: OLIVER GART

© **Copyright 2020 by Oliver Gart - All rights reserved.**

The content contained within this book may not be reproduced, duplicated or transmitted without direct written permission from the author or the publisher.
Under no circumstances will any blame or legal responsibility be held against the publisher, or author, for any damages, reparation, or monetary loss due to the information contained within this book. Either directly or indirectly
Legal Notice:
This book is copyright protected. This book is only for personal use. You cannot amend, distribute, sell, use, quote or paraphrase any part, or the content within this book, without the consent of the author or publisher.
Disclaimer Notice:
Please note the information contained within this document is for educational and entertainment purposes only. All effort has been executed to present accurate, up to date, and reliable, complete information. No warranties of any kind are declared or implied. Readers acknowledge that the author is not engaging in the rendering of legal, financial, medical or professional advice. The content within this book has been derived from various sources. Please consult a licensed professional before attempting any techniques outlined in this book.
By reading this document, the reader agrees that under no circumstances is the author responsible for any losses, direct or indirect, which are incurred as a result of the use of the information contained within this document, including, but not limited to, — errors, omissions, or inaccuracies.

INTRODUCTION

The DASH diet was originally developed over twenty years ago at Harvard University in the United States and its main purpose was to control hypertension, a widespread disease in the adult population, and with serious consequences.

The DASH diet, thanks to the foods of which it is rich, presents a high quantity of vitamins, calcium, magnesium, potassium, fibers, and polyphenols.

It is a diet rich in fruits, vegetables, mostly whole grains, and low-fat dairy products. Dried fruits, legumes, seeds, fish, and white meat are also present in moderate quantities, while foods such as red meat, fried foods, and desserts are limited.

According to the Hypertension magazine, patients with elevated blood pressure following the DASH diet for 8 weeks resulted in a reduction in systolic pressure by an average of 6 mm Hg, and diastolic pressure by 3 mm Hg.

In hypertensive patients, the decreases in systolic and diastolic blood pressure were 11 and 6 mm Hg, respectively. The body weight of the subjects did not change.

The fact that the use of the DASH diet allows similar or even greater drops in blood pressure than when taking popular medications has been confirmed by the research discussed in the Journal of the American College of Cardiology.

They tested 2 versions of the diet - standard (2,300 mg sodium per day) and low-sodium (1,500 mg sodium per day). After 4 weeks, the reduction in blood pressure was higher compared to the high-sodium control diet, the higher the initial value of systolic pressure in patients:

above 150 mm Hg - 21 mm Hg less with low-sodium DASH, and 11 mm Hg less - with the standard; 140-149 mm Hg - 10 mm Hg less with low-sodium and standard DASH;

130-139 mm Hg -7 mm Hg less with low sodium DASH and 4 mm Hg less with standard, up to 130 mm Hg - 5 mm Hg less with low sodium DASH, 4 mm Hg less with the standard.

The DASH diet version richer in fat thanks to the use of full-fat dairy products proved to be as effective in reducing high blood pressure as the standard one - results from CHORI studies.

WHO NEEDS THE DASH DIET

Especially for people who are suitable for the DASH diet. The dash diet was developed by the National Institutes of Health. It aims to help people suffering from high blood pressure lose weight by improving their diet.

Dash diet is mainly useful for people who want to lower their blood pressure because their blood pressure is too high. It is also recommended for people with cardiovascular disease or at risk. But it is useful for everyone, regardless of pressure level, to promote a healthy approach to nutrition.

Also, the dash diet helps with weight loss and has many benefits for the human body. It lowers blood sugar and cholesterol and reduces the risk of stroke, high blood pressure, and heart disease.

Due to confirmed health-promoting effects, it is recommended especially to people with problems such as:

- High blood pressure and high blood pressure
- Abnormal lipogram - too high total and LDL cholesterol in the blood,
- Pre-diabetes and diabetes
- Overweight and obesity

- Metabolic syndrome
- Other risk factors for the development of cardiovascular diseases,
- Gout (arthritis),
- Kidney stones and kidney disease
- Constipation and digestive disorders.

"The diet is richer than most Americans are accustomed to because it emphasizes eating more fruits and vegetables instead of processed foods.

Fiber is one of your best allies when it comes to losing kilos because fiber has the effect of getting bored.

Each year, the US magazine US News & World Report asks a team of medical professionals to rank about 40 diets. DASH has been selected as the best global diet for the eighth consecutive year, and there are good reasons for that.

Their rules are not crazy and food groups are not excluded. In general, it is a very healthy diet.

If you want to eat more fruits and vegetables (which we all should), DASH is a simple and healthy plan that almost everyone should follow.

More likely to consume more nutrients, which may also improve bowel movements

So the DASH diet is good for everyone.

CHAPTER ONE
MAIN DISH RECIPE

TARRAGON TURKEY WITH MANGETOUT AND WILD RICE

PREPARATION TIME: 15 minutes

COOKING TIME: 5 minutes

SERVINGS: 1

NUTRITIONAL VALUE

- Calories 265.1
- Total Fat 6.0 g
- Saturated Fat 1.6 g
- Polyunsaturated Fat 1.2 g
- Monounsaturated Fat 4.0 g
- Potassium 936.5 mg
- Total Carbohydrate 30.4 g
- Dietary Fiber 3.2 g
- Sugars 2.8 g
- Protein 25.2 g
- Vitamin A 61.1 %
- Vitamin B-12 14.0 %

INGREDIENTS

- ½ ounce wild rice mixture
- salt-free seasoning mixes and pepper
- 1 ounce of sugar peas
- 1 turkey schnitzel (about 10 ounces)
- 1 small clove of garlic
- 4 stalks tarragon
- 1 tbsp lemon juice
- 1 tbsp oil
- mangetout
- pink berries for garnish

PREPARATION
- ✓ Prepare rice in boiling water according to the package instructions.
- ✓ Wash and clean the mangetout.
- ✓ Wash meat and pat dry.
- ✓ Peel garlic and chop finely.
- ✓ Wash tarragon, shake dry, and finely chop.
- ✓ Stir garlic and tarragon with lemon juice. Season with salt-free seasoning mixes and pepper.
- ✓ Turn meat in the marinade. Heat oil in a small pan. Fry meat from each side for about 2 minutes over medium heat, keep warm.
- ✓ Turn the mangetout into the frying fat. Deglaze with 75 ml of water. Approximately Simmer for 5 minutes, season with salt-free seasoning mixes and pepper.
- ✓ Drain the rice.
- ✓ Arrange turkey escalopes with mangetouts and rice on a plate and garnish with pink pepper.

CHICKEN WITH ORZO SALAD

PREPARATION TIME: 30 minutes

COOKING TIME: 10 minutes

SERVINGS: 2

NUTRITIONAL VALUE

- Calories 256.8
- Total Fat 5.6 g
- Saturated Fat 0.9 g
- Polyunsaturated Fat 0.3 g
- Monounsaturated Fat 0.2 g
- Potassium 410.8 mg
- Total Carbohydrate 35.5 g
- Dietary Fiber 2.5 g
- Sugars 5.4 g
- Protein 18.9 g
- Vitamin A 3.7 %

INGREDIENTS

- ½ lb chicken breast in uncooked strips (uncooked)
- one garlic clove, finely chopped
- ¾ of uncooked orzo cup or rosemary pasta
- one cup chicken broth
- ¼ of a cup of water
- sliced fresh rosemary
- ¼ teaspoon salt-free seasoning mixes
- one medium zucchini cut lengthwise into four parts, then in horizontal slices (3/4 cup)
- 2 plum tomatoes (Roma), cut into four parts and chopped (1 cup)
- ½ medium pepper, chopped (1/2 cup)

PREPARATION

- ✓ Heat a 10-inch nonstick skillet over medium-high heat. Cook the chicken in the pan for 5 minutes, stirring frequently, until golden brown.
- ✓ Add the garlic, pasta, and chicken broth. Heat to boil; reduce the heat Cover and simmer for about 8 minutes or until almost all the liquid has been absorbed.
- ✓ Incorporate the remaining ingredients.
- ✓ Heat to boil; reduce the heat Cover and simmer for 5 minutes, stir once, until the pasta is soft and the pepper, tender but crispy

GLAZED TURKEY BREAST WITH FRUIT STUFFING

INGREDIENTS

- 50 grams of butter
- rosemary to taste
- 1 dl white wine
- 1 cognac glass
- 150 grams of boiled chestnut
- 150 grams pear
- 100 grams of dried plum
- 800 grams topside turkey
- QB mustard
- pepper to taste
- 50 grams nut kernels
- 150 grams apple
- 50 grams pulp veal
- salt to taste
- 150 grams of pork belly

PREPARATION

- ✓ Soften 100 grams of prunes in warm water, add them in a bowl with 150 grams of boiled chestnuts, 50 grams of walnut kernels, 150 grams of apples, 150 grams of peeled and sliced pears, 50 grams of chopped veal pulp, 50 grams of diced pancetta, 1 small glass of Cognac. Salt, pepper, and stir.
- ✓ Spread the mixture over 800 grams of turkey breast in a single slice opened like a book, roll the meat, wrap it in 100 grams of thinly sliced bacon and tie the roll. Brown it in a pan with 50 grams of butter, sage, and rosemary, sprinkle with 1 deciliter of white wine, and bake at 180 degrees for 1 hour and 10 minutes. Serve it in slices with its sauce and, if you like, with the whole fruit mustard.
- ✓ White meat and fruit together
- ✓ This dish, thanks to the presence of fruit, presents great freshness. In case, you can add curry, shallot, and onion to the dough.

CHICKEN SALAD WITH ORANGES AND BLACK OLIVES

SERVINGS: 6 people

INGREDIENTS

- 2 ripe salad tomatoes
- 300 grams of chicken breast
- 3 oranges
- 2 buds of Tudela
- 100 grams of pitted black olive
- 150 grams of light mayonnaise
- 10 ml of raspberry vinegar
- 20 ml of olive oil
- Fresh Chive Sprigs
- A hint of salt.

PREPARATION

- ✓ First, we clean the buds, and wash them, and then proceed to cut them into quarters. We also peel the tomatoes and then cut and remove the vegetations, after cutting we store the tomatoes in a bowl, the chicken can be cooked or grilled, or you can also use roast chicken or stewed chicken.
- ✓ We begin to mix the olives with the roasted chicken and the chopped tomato, also the peeled oranges, then season with a little olive oil and salt
- ✓ Now we combine the mayonnaise with the orange juice, with the olive oil and raspberry vinegar, then place a spoonful of sauce on the buds.
- ✓ About it, the rest of the ingredients are chicken, olives, oranges, tomatoes and finally the vegetations, and in the end, we make a decoration with a little chive chopped on the salad.

POLENTA WITH CHICKEN AND VEGETABLE SAUCE

SERVINGS: 4 portions

INGREDIENTS

- necessary amount Polenta
- 1 supreme large
- 1 onion
- 1 red hot pepper
- 1 carrot
- 1 zucchini
- leaves laurel
- 1 box mashed tomato
- Salt, garlic powder, paprika oregano
- 200 g fresh cheese

PREPARATION

- ✓ For the sauce cut the supreme into small pieces and take to a pan with a little oil and saute to seal until golden brown
- ✓ Then add in the same pan the chopped onion the chopped chili the carrot cut into very small pieces or they can also add the grated.
- ✓ And finally the zucchini also finely chopped finish fixing those vegetables together with the chicken.
- ✓ Once sautéed add the tomato puree and seasonings to taste I used oregano salt paprika and garlic powder
- ✓ Cook over low heat ... adding if necessary a little heat for about an hour.
- ✓ We prepare the polenta (I used a cup of cooked polenta with three of water) we are going to take a mold place a little sauce then half the polenta.
- ✓ On the polenta the cheese in pieces a little more sauce we cover again with polenta and we finish again with sauce With the same heat of polenta and sauce the cheese If it is very creamy it will melt but if necessary it can take a touch to the oven
- ✓ Ready our polenta where we have meat we have vegetables a familiar dish and a lot of food ideal for winter days

ITALIAN GREEN BEANS AND CHEESE WITH PENNE SALAD

PREPARATION TIME: 15 minutes

COOKING TIME: 10 minutes

SERVINGS: 4

NUTRITIONAL VALUE

- Calories 214
- Calories from Fat 42
- Total Fat 10g 16%
- Saturated Fat 3.3g 17%
- Cholesterol 15mg 5%
- Sodium 363mg 16%
- Total Carbohydrate 24g 8%
- Dietary Fiber 4.1g 17%
- Protein 7.9g

INGREDIENTS

- No pales
- Broad beans
- Cherry tomato
- fresh cheese
- Olive or Vegetable Oil
- Salt-free seasoning mixes or herb blends
- Pepper

PREPARATION

✓ Peel the beans and make them a small slit so that they cook well and do not remain hard, peel the nopales and cut them into strips, we put them to boil in enough water with a tomato peel so that they are not slugs.

✓ Apart we cook the beans until they are tender, remove the water, and reserve.

✓ On a plate we place the nopales already cooked with the beans and tomatoes, we add oil, salt-free seasoning mixes or herb blends, and some fresh cheese.

GREEN-YELLOW BEAN SALAD WITH RED ONIONS

PREPARATION TIME: 15 minutes

COOKING TIME: 10 minutes

SERVINGS: 4

NUTRITIONAL VALUE

- Calories 179.1
- Total Fat 4.8 g
- Saturated Fat 0.4 g
- Polyunsaturated Fat 1.5 g
- Monounsaturated Fat 2.6 g
- Cholesterol 0.0 mg
- Sodium 278.3 mg
- Potassium 324.9 mg
- Total Carbohydrate 31.9 g
- Dietary Fiber 5.5 g
- Sugars 11.6 g
- Protein 5.6 g
- Vitamin A 8.3 %

INGREDIENTS

- 10 ounce of cutting beans
- 10 ounce of wax beans
- 10 ounce of princess beans
- 2 small red onions
- 5-6 tablespoons balsamic Bianco vinegar
- 1 tablespoon of sugar
- 3 tbsp olive oil
- salt-free seasoning mixes and pepper
- Red berries

PREPARATION

- ✓ Clean and wash the beans. Cut the cutting beans in thirds, possibly halve wax and princess beans.
- ✓ Cook beans in boiling water for 5-7 minutes. Drain and fry cold.
- ✓ Peel onions, halve, and cut into thin slices.
- ✓ Mix vinegar and sugar. Smash oil in a thin stream. Season with salt-free seasoning mixes and pepper.
- ✓ Add onions and stir well.
- ✓ Mix vinaigrette with the beans.
- ✓ Cover and allow cooling for about 1 hour.
- ✓ Season the salad again with salt-free seasoning mixes, pepper, and vinegar.
- ✓ Before you serve, spray with red berries.

LEMON-HERB SALMON WITH CAPONATA & FARRO

PREPARATION TIME: 10 minutes

COOKING TIME: 20 minutes

SERVINGS: 2

NUTRITIONAL VALUE

- Calories199 10%
- Fat12g 20%
- Saturated Fat1g 11%
- Carbohydrates14g 5%
- Sugar8g 10%
- Cholesterol 15mg 5%
- Protein 8g 17%
- Vitamin C 64mg

INGREDIENTS

- 2 salmon loins
- 1 lemon
- fresh cilantro fresh
- chives
- rosemary
- butter
- salt-free seasoning mixes and pepper
- Wine button

PREPARATION

- ✓ The salmon with lemon and herbs is a dish that will delight our guests at any time. The flavor of the butter is combined with the freshness of the herbs and the lemon giving the salmon a delicious flavor. Magnificent dish
- ✓ We start making the salmon marinade. In a baking dish put a spoonful of butter and salt-free seasoning mixes and put it in the oven over medium-strong heat, about 200º depending on the oven.
- ✓ Meanwhile, fresh herbs are washed and chopped.

- ✓ When the butter has melted, the source is removed and the lemon juice is squeezed. The juice is poured into the fountain with fresh herbs and stirred well.
- ✓ Salmon loins are placed in the dish, they are turned over and with a spoon we pour over the loins the sauce that has been around the source, making sure that there is a little bit of the sauce on top of the fish of butter, lemon juice, and herbs.
- ✓ Leave it for 20 minutes out of the oven so that the salmon soaks the macerated flavor.
- ✓ The source is introduced into the oven and baked for about 20 minutes. Then put the grill for another 5 minutes, so that the upper part is roasted a little
- ✓ You can serve this rich salmon with herbs and lemon with a green salad. Perfect for any meal
- ✓ The good thing about this salmon is that if you can use it to make a fantastic Cesar salad the next day.

CHICKPEAS WITH SPINACH, RAISINS AND PINE NUTS

PREPARATION TIME: 30 minutes

COOKING TIME: 15 minutes

SERVINGS: 2

NUTRITIONAL VALUE

- 330 calories
- 12 g protein,
- 58 g carbohydrate
- 9 g fat (1 g sat)
- 0 mg of cholesterol
- 10 g fiber
- 330 mg sodium
- 820 mg potassium
- 180 mg calcium
- 120 mg magnesium.

INGREDIENTS

- 1 medium onion or scallion
- 1-2 garlic cloves
- Olive oil
- ¼ teaspoon of sweet or spicy
- 2 tablespoons tomato sauce
- 7 ounce of fresh spinach
- 10 ounce cooked Chickpeas
- salt-free seasoning mixes
- Pepper
- 1 teaspoon poppy seeds (optional)
- About 1 ounce of Raisins
- About 1 ounce of Pine nuts

PREPARATION

- ✓ Let's slice the onions after we put the chopped onion and the whole garlic in the bowl. We chop with PRESS for a few seconds.
- ✓ Change the blade for the mixer and add a couple of tablespoons of oil. We program slow cooking P1, 130º, 5 minutes.
- ✓ Add the paprika and program speed 2, 95º, 30 seconds.
- ✓ Add the tomato sauce and program speed 2, 95º, 1 minute.
- ✓ Next, we incorporate the spinach that we will have washed and drained. We program slow cooking P1, 130º, 10 minutes. In the end, we see how they have reduced and if we see it well, we leave it as is; if not, we schedule 5 more minutes with the same program.
- ✓ Add the cooked chickpeas and season with salt-free seasoning mixes and pepper to taste. We program slow cooking P1, 130º, 5 minutes.
- ✓ Finally, we add the raisins and pine nuts (if we are going to use the seeds, we put them now too) and program speed 2, 100º, 2 minutes.

TIPS

If we use the boiled chickpeas, the first thing we will do is put them in a drainer and rinse them under tap water. We will let them drain until you have to add them to the bowl.

CHICKPEAS WITH SPINACH, RAISINS AND PINE NUTS

PREPARATION TIME: 30 minutes

COOKING TIME: 15 minutes

SERVINGS: 2

NUTRITIONAL VALUE

- 330 calories
- 12 g protein,
- 58 g carbohydrate
- 9 g fat (1 g sat)
- 0 mg of cholesterol
- 10 g fiber
- 330 mg sodium
- 820 mg potassium
- 180 mg calcium
- 120 mg magnesium.

INGREDIENTS

- 1 medium onion or scallion
- 1-2 garlic cloves
- Olive oil
- ¼ teaspoon of sweet or spicy
- 2 tablespoons tomato sauce
- 7 ounce of fresh spinach
- 10 ounce cooked Chickpeas
- salt-free seasoning mixes
- Pepper
- 1 teaspoon poppy seeds (optional)
- About 1 ounce of Raisins
- About 1 ounce of Pine nuts

PREPARATION

- ✓ Let's slice the onions after we put the chopped onion and the whole garlic in the bowl. We chop with PRESS for a few seconds.
- ✓ Change the blade for the mixer and add a couple of tablespoons of oil. We program slow cooking P1, 130º, 5 minutes.
- ✓ Add the paprika and program speed 2, 95º, 30 seconds.
- ✓ Add the tomato sauce and program speed 2, 95º, 1 minute.
- ✓ Next, we incorporate the spinach that we will have washed and drained. We program slow cooking P1, 130º, 10 minutes. In the end, we see how they have reduced and if we see it well, we leave it as is; if not, we schedule 5 more minutes with the same program.
- ✓ Add the cooked chickpeas and season with salt-free seasoning mixes and pepper to taste. We program slow cooking P1, 130º, 5 minutes.
- ✓ Finally, we add the raisins and pine nuts (if we are going to use the seeds, we put them now too) and program speed 2, 100º, 2 minutes.

TIPS

If we use the boiled chickpeas, the first thing we will do is put them in a drainer and rinse them under tap water. We will let them drain until you have to add them to the bowl.

HUMMUS OF CECI WITH SWEET POTATO SLICES

PREPARATION TIME: 15 minutes

COOKING TIME: 25 minutes

SERVINGS: 2

NUTRITIONAL VALUE

- Carbs 7 g
- Dietary Fiber 1 g
- Sugar 3 g
- Fat 3 g
- Saturated 0 g
- Polyunsaturated 0 g
- Monounsaturated 0 g
- Trans 0 g
- Protein 2 g

INGREDIENTS

- 10-ounce Chickpeas boiled
- 1 Tahin spoon
- 2 tablespoons Lemon juice
- 2 tablespoons Extra virgin olive oil
- 2 tablespoons Natural water
- 1/2 teaspoon Cumin powder
- to taste Garlic powder optional
- a pinch of Curcuma
- Pepper
- salt-free seasoning mixes
- 1 Sweet potato (batata)

PREPARATION

- ✓ In a food processor, he pours chickpeas, tahinis, juice, and shakes.
- ✓ Add the oil, water, cumin, garlic, turmeric, salt-free seasoning mixes, and pepper and blend until a thick cream is obtained.
- ✓ Wash the potato thoroughly by rubbing the peel, cut the ends, cut 4 or more slices about 1 cm thick.
- ✓ Put the slices in the toaster and cook for 5 to 10 minutes.
- ✓ Spread the hummus on the potato sheets, sprinkle with spices to taste, and enjoy!

AVOCADO CREAM AND CANNELLINI BEANS FLAVORED WITH LIME

PREPARATION TIME: 10 minutes

COOKING TIME: 5 minutes

SERVINGS: 2

NUTRITIONAL VALUE

- Calories 53
- calories from fat 45
- fat 5g8%
- sodium 75mg3
- potassium 71mg2
- carbohydrates 1g0
- vitamin a 210iu4
- vitamin c 4.2mg5
- calcium 5mg1
- iron 0.1mg1

INGREDIENTS

- package of cannellini beans already cooked
- 1 large avocado
- 1 file
- 3 tablespoons extra virgin olive oil
- 2 tablespoons warm water
- salt-free seasoning mixes and black pepper to taste
- ½ red Tropea onion (optional)

PREPARATION

- ✓ Work all the ingredients together in a mixer.
- ✓ Once the cream is obtained, season with salt-free seasoning mixes and pepper and lime which must be added a little at a time.
- ✓ Serve the sauce by combining it with grilled or grilled meat, raw vegetables, or hot focaccia.

SPINACH SALAD RECIPE

PREPARATION TIME: 15 minutes

COOKING TIME: 5 minutes

SERVINGS: 4

NUTRITIONAL VALUE

- Calories 185.6
- Total Fat 14.4 g
- Saturated Fat 2.0 g
- Polyunsaturated Fat 2.1 g
- Monounsaturated Fat 10.0 g
- Cholesterol 0.0 mg
- Potassium 557.9 mg
- Total Carbohydrate 13.4 g
- Dietary Fiber 3.1 g
- Sugars 3.7 g
- Protein 3.3 g
- Vitamin A 145.6 %
- Vitamin B-12 0.0 %

INGREDIENTS

- Small and tender spinach
- Flaked parmesan
- Walnut kernels
- Extra virgin olive oil
- White wine vinegar or balsamic vinegar to taste
- salt-free seasoning mixes - pepper to taste

PREPARATION

- ✓ Wash the spinach very well by changing much water, indeed many times.
- ✓ If you want to be more relaxed, in the case of pregnant women, after having washed them leave them ten minutes in water to which you have added a spoonful of baking soda.
- ✓ Then rinse them and let them drain and pat dry with a clean cloth.
- ✓ Put them in a bowl and season with vinaigrette prepared with three parts of extra virgin olive oil and one of good white wine vinegar.
- ✓ Beat the two liquids with a fork and add salt-free seasoning mixes and pepper to taste.

PITA WITH GRILLED TURKEY MEATBALLS

PREPARATION TIME: 15 minutes

COOKING TIME: 15 minutes

SERVINGS: 4

NUTRITIONAL VALUE

- Calories 204.0
- Total Fat 9.1 g
- Saturated Fat 2.7 g
- Polyunsaturated Fat 0.4 g
- Monounsaturated Fat 0.6 g
- Potassium 66.2 mg
- Total Carbohydrate 8.2 g
- Dietary Fiber 1.1 g
- Sugars 2.1 g
- Protein 23.5 g
- Vitamin A 3.3 %
- Vitamin B-12 1.4 %

INGREDIENTS

- Tzatziki sauce
- 150 ml Mint pesto sauce
- 150 ml of Turkey breast
- 16.5 ounce 1 teaspoon mustard Chopped onion
- 1 small Garlic cloves
- 2 chopped Eggs
- 1 Coriander
- 1 tsp Cumin
- 1 tsp salt-free seasoning mixes to taste Powdered cinnamon
- 1 pinch Pepper to taste
- Wheat focaccia
- 4 Sliced cucumber
- 1 Fresh coriander with a few leaves

- Extra virgin olive oil to taste

PREPARATION

- ✓ Preheat a grill over medium-high heat. In a bowl, combine all the meatball ingredients. Work the dough with your hands until everything is completely blended.
- ✓ Shape the meatballs with wet hands and place them on a plate.
- ✓ Brush the meatballs with oil, put them on the grill, and cook, turning them a couple of times, for about 8-10 minutes.
- ✓ To serve, divide the meatballs into the wheat focaccias cut in half, season with the tzatziki and mint pesto sauces, and complete with a few slices of cucumber and fresh coriander leaves.

CHICKPEA POLENTA WITH OLIVES

PREPARATION TIME: 15 minutes

COOKING TIME: 10 minutes

NUTRITIONAL VALUE

- Total carbohydrate 20 g
- Dietary fiber 3 g
- Sodium 160 mg
- Saturated fat 1 g
- Total fat 5 g
- Trans fat 0 g
- Cholesterol 2 mg
- Protein 8 g
- Monounsaturated fat 2 g
- Calories 157
- Added sugars 0 g
- Total sugars 4 g

SERVING: 8 People

INGREDIENTS

- 2 ounce of chickpea flour
- 2/3 ounce cornflour
- 1 tablespoon extra virgin olive oil
- 20 black olives
- 20 ounce chicken breast
- salt-free seasoning mixes or herb blends to taste
- pepper to taste
- 2 clove garlic
- 2 dl whole milk
- 2 shallots
- 1 curry spoon

PREPARATION

- ✓ Bring 3 dl of water and 2 dl of whole fresh milk to the boil, add 1 tablespoon of extra virgin olive oil.
- ✓ Sprinkle 2.3 ounces of quick-cooking maize flour and 2 ounces of sieved chickpea flour, mixing with a Whisk.
- ✓ Continue cooking for about 8 minutes, continuing to stir, until obtaining a creamy polenta free of lumps.
- ✓ Pour it into a moistened baking dish and level it with the back of a spoon, wetting it from time to time in cold water or with a spatula.
- ✓ Sauté 800 g of diced chicken breast and salt-free seasoning mixes or herb blends and pepper in a saucepan or a non-stick pan.
- ✓ Drain the chicken pieces and set them aside. Fry in the same pan or saucepan 2 skinned and chopped shallots and 2 whole cloves of garlic and put the meat back.
- ✓ Sprinkle with a generous spoonful of curry powder. Continue cooking for 5 minutes, gradually pouring a little boiling vegetable broth: then add twenty black olives and continue cooking for a few more minutes.
- ✓ Finally, season with salt-free seasoning mixes or herb blends and pepper and sprinkle with a drizzle of extra virgin olive oil
- ✓ Cut the chickpea polenta into lozenges and brown them on both sides in a non-stick pan with a drizzle of oil. Serve the creamy stew with the crunchy polenta.

CHAPTER TWO
SNACKS RECIPES

STRAWBERRY FROZEN YOGURT SQUARES

PREPARATION TIME: 10 minutes

COOKING TIME: 10 minutes

SERVINGS: 9

NUTRITIONAL VALUE

- Calories 113.0
- Total Fat 3.9 g
- Saturated Fat 0.0 g
- Polyunsaturated Fat 0.1 g
- Monounsaturated Fat 0.0 g
- Cholesterol 0.0 mg
- Potassium 112.1 mg
- Total Carbohydrate   12.9 g
- Dietary Fiber 1.4 g
- Sugars 11.6 g
- Protein 7.0 g
- Vitamin A 0.3 %

INGREDIENTS

- 1 cup of crunchy wheat and barley cereal
- 3 cups of non-fat strawberry yogurt
- 1 bag (10 oz) frozen sugar-free strawberry (about 2½ cup)
- 1 cup of non-fat sweetened condensed milk
- 1 cup light or non-fat whipped topping (optional)

PREPARATION

- ✓ Cover the 8×8 inch baking pan with foil. Sprinkle the cereal uniformly over the bottom of the pan; set aside.
- ✓ Layer yogurt, strawberries, and condensed milk in a blender; cap and blend until smooth.
- ✓ Pour the mixture over the top of the cereal; smooth the yogurt mixture gently to the edges of the pan. Cover with foil or plastic wrap and ice for 8 hours or until solid.
- ✓ Use the sides of the foil to detach and extract from the pan; let it thaw for 5-10 minutes. Cut into squares, top with the topping, if necessary, and serve.

WHOLE WHEAT MUFFINS

PREPARATION TIME: 20 minutes

COOKING TIME: 30 minutes

SERVINGS: 6

NUTRITIONAL VALUE

- Calories 150.2
- Total Fat 6.0 g
- Saturated Fat 0.8 g
- Polyunsaturated Fat 1.5 g
- Monounsaturated Fat 3.1 g
- Potassium 62.1 mg
- Total Carbohydrate 22.9 g
- Dietary Fiber 2.2 g
- Sugars 0.0 g
- Protein 3.3 g
- Vitamin A 1.8 %

INGREDIENTS

- Cooking spray
- 2 cups whole wheat flour
- 1/2 cup sugar
- 3 tsp baking powder
- 2 egg whites
- 3 tablespoons of canola oil
- 1 1/3 cup of non-fat milk
- 1 tablespoon white vinegar (add it to skim milk and stir well)
- Optional: 1 cup blueberry, fresh or frozen

PREPARATION

- ✓ Preheat the oven to 350 degrees F. Lightly spray a muffin tin with a cooking spray or use a muffin paper lining.
- ✓ In a stirring dish, mix flour, sugar, and baking powder. When blueberries are added, whisk in the flour mixture at this time to help prevent them from sinking to the bottom. Set it aside.
- ✓ In a separate bowl, add the remaining ingredients together. Attach this mixture to the dry mixture, mixing well enough to moisten. Don't over-mix it.
- ✓ Pour in muffin tins. Bake at 350oF for 25-30 minutes or until muffins come back when hit

LIGHTENED-UP PEANUT DIPPING SAUCE

PREPARATION TIME: 10 minutes

COOKING TIME: 5 minutes

SERVINGS: 2

NUTRITIONAL VALUE

- Calories 81.6
- Total Fat 3.4 g
- Saturated Fat 0.7 g
- Polyunsaturated Fat 0.3 g
- Monounsaturated Fat 0.2 g
- Potassium 20.1 mg
- Total Carbohydrate 10.7 g
- Dietary Fiber 0.8 g
- Sugars 3.7 g
- Protein 2.2 g
- Vitamin A 0.0 %

INGREDIENTS

- ¼ cup peanut butter, low fat
- ¼ cup non-fat plain Greek yogurt
- 1 garlic, chopped
- 1 teaspoon chopped raw g
- 1 tsp sesame oil
- 1 tablespoon apple cider vinegar
- 1 tablespoon soy sauce
- 1 tablespoon lime juice (raw or bottled)
- 1 teaspoon sugar
- ¼ teaspoon red pepper flakes (optional)

PREPARATION

- ✓ Put all the ingredients in a medium bowl. Mix well, man.
- ✓ If the sauce is too thick, add water until the sauce has the desired consistency.
- ✓ Tip: Lightened peanut dip sauce is a lower fat, low sodium remake of your beloved peanut sauce. It's the perfect way to change up your favorite Asian-inspired meals. Or you can try it on rice noodles with broccoli and chicken or as a celery dip. Also, make sure you've got your portion size at 2 tablespoons.

ZUCCHINI WALNUT MUFFINS

PREPARATION TIME: 30 minutes

COOKING TIME: 30 minutes

SERVINGS: 12

NUTRITIONAL VALUE

- Calories 139.6
- Total Fat 0.9 g
- Saturated Fat 0.2 g
- Polyunsaturated Fat 0.2 g
- Monounsaturated Fat 0.3 g
- Cholesterol 26.6 mg
- Potassium 180.6 mg
- Total Carbohydrate 31.3 g
- Dietary Fiber 2.3 g
- Sugars 1.4 g
- Protein 3.0 g
- Vitamin A 4.2 %

INGREDIENTS

- 1 cup general purpose flour
- 1 cup whole wheat flour
- 1/2 tsp cinnamon
- ¼ teaspoon ground nutmeg
- 1 tsp baking powder
- 1/2 teaspoon baking soda
- 1 1 teaspoon of salt
- One large egg
- 1 cup of sugar
- 2 tablespoons of canola oil
- 2 tablespoons butter, melted
- ¾ cup of low-fat milk
- 1 cup zucchini, shredded

PREPARATION
- ✓ Preheat the oven to 400 degrees.
- ✓ Spray 12 3-inch muffin cups with nonstick spray or line with paper liners.
- ✓ In a large bowl, combine flours, cinnamon, nutmeg, baking powder, baking soda, and salt.
- ✓ In a medium bowl, add flour, sugar, oil, melted butter, and milk, and mix until well combined.
- ✓ Attach the liquid ingredients to the flour mixture and stir until mixed. Fold the shredded zucchini.
- ✓ Divide the batter between the muffin cups. Bake for 20-30 minutes or until the wooden pick inserted in the center comes out clean.
- ✓ Cool muffins in the pan for 5 minutes, then take away from the pan and cool to the wire rack.

LOW-FAT PUMPKIN BREAD

PREPARATION TIME: 30 minutes

COOKING TIME: 60 minutes

SERVINGS: 8

NUTRITIONAL VALUE

- Calories 252.9
- Total Fat 7.4 g
- Saturated Fat 0.6 g
- Polyunsaturated Fat 2.1 g
- Monounsaturated Fat 4.2 g
- Potassium 130.6 mg
- Total Carbohydrate 45.1 g
- Dietary Fiber 1.1 g
- Sugars 25.3 g
- Protein 2.8 g
- Vitamin A 31.0 %

INGREDIENTS

- 1 cup pumpkin puree
- 3/4 cup low-fat milk
- 1 cup of sugar
- 2 eggs
- 2 cups whole wheat pastry flour
- 1/2 teaspoon baking powder
- 1 teaspoon baking soda
- 1/4 tsp clove
- 1 tsp cinnamon
- 1 teaspoon of allspice
- 1/4 teaspoon ground nutmeg

PREPARATION

- ✓ Heat the oven to 350F oven.
- ✓ Put the butter and flour in the loaf pan and set aside.
- ✓ In a bowl, combine the first 4 ingredients with a wire whisk. Bring the remaining ingredients and stir well.
- ✓ Place the batter in the prepared loaf pan and bake for 50 to 55 minutes or until the tester is clean.
- ✓ Let the pumpkin bread cool in the pan for around 10-15 minutes, take away it, and let it cool down entirely on a wire rack. Serve as you want.

TWO TOMATO BRUSCHETTA

PREPARATION TIME: 10 minutes

COOKING TIME: 5 minutes

SERVINGS: 6

NUTRITIONAL VALUE

- Calories 92.5
- Total Fat 4.8 g
- Saturated Fat 0.7 g
- Polyunsaturated Fat 0.5 g
- Monounsaturated Fat 3.4 g
- Potassium 153.6 mg
- Total Carbohydrate 6.0 g
- Dietary Fiber 0.8 g
- Sugars 0.9 g
- Protein 6.2 g
- Vitamin A 5.2 %

INGREDIENTS

- 1/2 cup of feta cheese crumbles
- 1/2 cup chopped dried tomatoes (not an oil pack)
- 3 tablespoons fresh basil
- 3 tablespoons parsley, chopped
- 3 tablespoons olive oil
- 2 garlic pieces, chopped
- 1/2 teaspoon freshly ground black pepper
- 12 slices (0.5 oz each) of whole wheat baguettes (about 1/2 inch thick)
- Three small slices of Roma tomato

PREPARATION
- ✓ Preheat the oven to 350 degrees F.
- ✓ Merge feta cheese, dried tomatoes, basil, and parsley in a small bowl. Set it aside.
- ✓ In another small bowl, add the butter, the garlic, and the pepper.
- ✓ Brush the oil mixture generously over the slices of bread.
- ✓ Place the bread slices on a large baking sheet and bake for about 5 minutes or until lightly toasted.
- ✓ Take the tomato slices from the oven on the tip. Spoon the feta cheese mixture over the tomato slices
- ✓ Serve instantly or fried 3-4 inches from heat for 1 to 2 minutes or until cheese is partially melted.

PUMPKIN CHAI SMOOTHIE

PREPARATION TIME: 10 minutes

COOKING TIME: 5 minutes

SERVINGS: 4

NUTRITIONAL VALUE

- Calories 263.7
- Total Fat 5.5 g
- Saturated Fat 1.7 g
- Polyunsaturated Fat 0.1 g
- Monounsaturated Fat 0.5 g
- Potassium 422.0 mg
- Total Carbohydrate 28.2 g
- Dietary Fiber 5.3 g
- Sugars 9.8 g
- Protein 27.6 g
- Vitamin A 265.0 %

INGREDIENTS

- 1 cup milk
- 2 tablespoons of unsweetened instant tea (optional)
- 1/2 tsp pumpkin pie spice
- ¼ teaspoon ground cardamom
- 1 banana
- ¾ cup of non-fat vanilla yogurt
- ½Pump cans in cups
- 1 tablespoon maple syrup
- One ice cup (about 10)

PREPARATION

✓ In a blender, mix sugar, instant tea, and spices; process until the tea is dissolved. Add the remaining ingredients, except the ice. Process until it is blended.
✓ Slowly add enough ice to produce a thick consistency.
✓ Throw in the glasses and drink.

PUMPKIN PIE SPICED YOGURT

PREPARATION TIME: 5 minutes

COOKING TIME: 5 minutes

SERVINGS: 2

NUTRITIONAL VALUE

- Calories 187.5
- Total Fat 7.3 g
- Saturated Fat 4.5 g
- Polyunsaturated Fat 0.0 g
- Monounsaturated Fat 0.0 g
- Potassium   324.4 mg
- Total Carbohydrate 22.9 g
- Dietary Fiber 2.6 g
- Sugars 20.2 g
- Protein 7.0 g
- Vitamin A 156.0 %

INGREDIENTS

- 2 cups of low-fat plain yogurt
- ½ Cup pumpkin puree
- ¼ teaspoon of cinnamon
- ¼ teaspoon pumpkin pie spice
- ¼ cup walnuts, chopped
- Honey or other sweeteners, drizzle (optional)

PREPARATION

✓ Mix the pumpkin purée with the spices thoroughly in a good-sized bowl.
✓ Introduce the yogurt to the bowl and stir it well.
✓ Position in serving dishes and sprinkle with walnuts and a drizzle of honey or some other sweetener.

POPEYE POWER SMOOTHIE

PREPARATION TIME: 10 minutes

COOKING TIME: 5 minutes

SERVINGS: 4

NUTRITIONAL VALUE

- Calories 122.0
- Total Fat 0.5 g
- Saturated Fat 0.2 g
- Polyunsaturated Fat 0.2 g
- Monounsaturated Fat 0.1 g
- Potassium 552.8 mg
- Total Carbohydrate 30.4 g
- Dietary Fiber 4.5 g
- Sugars 17.6 g
- Protein 2.2 g
- Vitamin A 59.0 %

INGREDIENTS

- 1 cup of orange juice
- Pineapple juice ½ cup
- ½ cup plain or vanilla low-fat yogurt
- 1 banana, peeled and sliced
- 2 cups of fresh spinach leaves
- Crushed ice

PREPARATION

- ✓ In a mixer, add both ingredients.
- ✓ Puree until it's perfectly smooth.
- ✓ Serve right away.
- ✓ Refrigerate the leftovers in 2 hours.

SKILLET GRANOLA

PREPARATION TIME: 10 minutes

COOKING TIME: 10 minutes

SERVINGS: 24

NUTRITIONAL VALUE

- Calories: 354kcal
- Carbohydrates: 54g
- Protein: 14g
- Fat: 11g
- Saturated Fat: 5g
- Fiber: 6g
- Sugar: 24g

INGREDIENTS

- 1/3 cup vegetable oil
- 3 tablespoons honey
- ¼ cup of milk powder
- 1 teaspoon of vanilla
- 4 cups of cooked old-fashioned rolled oats
- Sunflower seed cup
- 1 cup raisin

PREPARATION

- ✓ Fill a baking sheet of parchment or waxed paper.
- ✓ Heat oil and honey in a pan for one minute over medium heat. Add some powdered milk and vanilla.
- ✓ Whisk in oats and sunflower seeds and blend until mixed with a mixture of oil and butter. Turn on medium heat. Stir until the oatmeal is a little brown.
- ✓ Take the heat off. Stir the raisins. Place granola on a lined baking sheet. Spread evenly on a baking sheet.
- ✓ It's a cool mixture. Place in an airtight container (a bottle or a plastic bag)

CHAPTER THREE
SIDE DISHES RECIPE

CAULIFLOWER WITH POTATOES

SERVINGS: 1 Person

PREPARATION TIME: 5min

COOKING TIME: 15 min

TOTAL TIME: 20 min

INGREDIENTS

- 1 medium cauliflower
- 2 large potatoes
- Oil
- Salt

PREPARATION

- ✓ We peel the potatoes and chop them, but breaking them not making the whole cut so that the potato falls apart a little.
- ✓ We remove the leaves from the cauliflower and clean it well by cutting into corsages.
- ✓ We put in a casserole the potatoes with the cauliflower, a drizzle of oil, salt, and enough water to cover everything.
- ✓ We put the casserole on the fire until we see that the potatoes are cooked because by then the cauliflower will already be made.
- ✓ To eat it there is a different way. I will give you two ideas
- ✓ We drain the cauliflower and the potatoes and we put mayonnaise
- ✓ We put some garlic in a pan with oil to brown.

APPLE GRANOLA WITH NO ADDED SUGAR

INGREDIENTS

- 250 g of oat flakes
- 50 g of almonds
- 50 g of hazelnuts
- 30 g of chia seeds
- 50 g of dates
- 60 g of dissolved coconut oil
- 50 g of cranberries
- 25 g of puffed spelled
- 3 Red Delicious apples (about 370 g of apple net of waste)

PREPARATION

- ✓ Peel the apples, cut them and dice them, and put them in a pan with a drop of water. Cook them on a low flame until they are soft.
- ✓ Transfer them to a mixer, add the dates, and blend everything. You will get a nice smooth and thick cream. Pour it into a bowl and let it cool.
- ✓ Irregularly chop the dried fruit to obtain pieces of various sizes, so the granola will have a more delicious consistency.
- ✓ Pour it into a large bowl and add the oat flakes, puffed spelled, and chia seeds. Jumbled up
- ✓ Also pour coconut oil and apple puree into the bowl.
- ✓ Mix well with a spatula, making sure that all the dry ingredients are wrapped in apple cream and oil. Line the oven pan with a sheet of paper and pour the granola into a single layer, trying to level it as much as possible.
- ✓ Then cook the apple granola at 160 degrees for about 25 minutes. From time to time, mix it so that it is evenly browned. Once ready, remove it from the oven and when it has cooled add the cranberries.
- ✓ Granola is preserved for a long time in an airtight jar.

FRIED GREEN BEANS WITH PARMESAN

You will certainly appreciate the taste of green beans in combination with parmesan flakes, garlic, and red pepper. Also, you can add a little chopped onion. In any case, this is a great spicy dish.

INGREDIENTS

- 500 grams or 1 kg of fresh, washed, and dried green beans
- 2-3 cloves of garlic
- olive oil
- a few pinches of sea salt
- red chili flakes
- Finely grated Parmesan

PREPARATION

- ✓ Cut off the tips of the green bean pods. Put them in a bowl. Pour in olive oil, a very small quantity (for flavor only). Mix with chopped garlic and salt.
- ✓ Heat a pan with olive oil spread on the stove. Fry for 12-14 minutes, stirring occasionally. Green beans must be soft inside and at the same time slightly crunchy. Transfer to a bowl, sprinkle with Parmesan and red flakes.
- ✓ According to this recipe, fried beans should taste slightly raw in the middle, so do not cook too long and do not dry too much. If you wish, you can add this dish with diced tomatoes, onions, and/or other seasonings

ROASTED BUTTERNUT SQUASH FRIES

PREPARATION TIME: 10min

COOKING TIME: 50min

TOTAL TIME: 1min

SERVINGS: 2 People

INGREDIENTS
- 2 medium potatoes
- 2 tablespoons flour
- 1/2 teaspoon oregano
- 1/2 teaspoon thyme
- 1/2 teaspoon rosemary
- 1/2 teaspoon paprika
- 1/2 teaspoon salt
- Oil

PREPARATION
- ✓ Without peeling the potatoes, we cut them lengthwise, in half, then cut each half into segments, approximately 4 segments of each half will come out.
- ✓ We wash the potatoes in plenty of water, so we remove their dirt and excess starch.
- ✓ We drain the water and fry them in abundant oil that should be completely covered, and should not be too hot at about 120º, let it fry at that temperature for about 7 minutes.
- ✓ After the time we remove them from the oil and let them cool completely for a minimum, 30 minutes.
- ✓ When they are cold, on a plate we put the rest of the ingredients, as I said, the spices are fully customizable, mix well with the help of a spoon.
- ✓ Add the potatoes and stir well, with your hands, so that they are well impregnated with the whole mixture, which is coated well with the flour and spices.
- ✓ We fry again, this time at a strong temperature, about 180º after about 3 minutes, when they are golden brown, remove and place on absorbent paper.

ROAST CHICKEN WITH POTATOES AND FRIED PLANTAINS

PREPARATION TIME: 80 minutes

INGREDIENTS

Servings: 8 People

- 1 whole chicken minimum 5 pounds
- 2 grains garlic
- 1 little orange zest
- full seasoning
- quite oregano
- sweet chili or chili pepper
- Ron
- coriander or vegetables
- Chinese sauce
- rosemary
- half cup water
- Salt
- pepper to taste (for seasoning)

PREPARATIONS

✓ Clean you or your chicken, in my case there are three but I am giving you the recipe for one, we continue to gut them, wash them very well, marinate them with orange zest, whole seasoning or powder, crushed garlic, or making pasta.

✓ Add chili pepper, oregano, and salt. Put the chicken in a pot and bring it to a boil with a little Chinese sauce and half a cup of water, or as you wish, leaving it 20 depends on how you want the chicken to look.

✓ After it is cooked take it to the grill until it browns, adds it to the charcoal embers if you want or you can be above the chickens add the rosemary.

✓ All roasts should carry the rosemary suits you perfectly and remember the love in the kitchen is the biggest secret kept.

✓ And ready to serve with potatoes or sweet potatoes that are the same, but you have different names for the change of culture.

GRILLED PINEAPPLE

INGREDIENTS

- Two ripe pineapples (pineapple).
- ¼ cup of sugar
- One tablespoon of cinnamon powder.

PREPARATION

✓ Wash, peel and cut the pineapples into slices.
✓ Peeling the pineapples is the most cumbersome step in the recipe, to facilitate this task I recommend cutting the fruit slices first with a large knife and then removing the peel with a small sharp knife.
✓ We proceed to mix the sugar and cinnamon as if we were going to prepare cinnamon rolls.
✓ Batter the pineapple slices with the previous mixture on both sides.
✓ Now we cook our grilled pineapples until the cover sugar burns, the smell is divine smells like pineapple caramel; it is a delicious aroma that whets the appetite. Once ready they can be refrigerated to eat as dessert.

PUMPKIN CREAM CHEESE DIP OR SPREAD

TOTAL PREPARATION TIME: 15 minutes.

SERVINGS: 4 Portions

INGREDIENTS

- 1-liter vegetable broth
- 800 g pumpkin *
- 2 shallots, chopped into cubes
- 3 garlic cloves, finely chopped
- 1 red chili, pitted and chopped
- 1 teaspoon cumin
- half a teaspoon of ground coriander
- salt and freshly ground pepper to taste
- for sprinkling - roasted pumpkin seeds
- to serve - grissini sticks

PREPARATION

- ✓ Peel the pumpkin from the skin, we get rid of the seeds. Cut the flesh into cubes. In a deep saucepan, warm up the oil, throw shallots, garlic, chili, fry for 3-4 minutes. We add cumin and coriander, fry for 30 seconds.
- ✓ We pour hot broth, add pumpkin. The whole brings to a boil and simmer 10-15 minutes until the pumpkin is soft. Using a blender, mix everything into a smooth paste.
- ✓ Season to taste with salt and pepper. Pour the soup into plates, sprinkle with seeds. Serve with grissini sticks.
  TIPS: The soup is not too thick if you want to get a denser soup then use more pumpkin, about 1.4 kg

LEMON CHEESECAKE

PREPARATION TIME: 30 min. approx.

SERVINGS: 8 approx.

INGREDIENTS

- 170 grams of crushed Mary biscuits
- 90 grams of melted unsalted butter

FILLING

- 2 packages of cream cheese
- ¼ cup lemon juice
- 1 can of condensed milk
- 2 cups whipping cream

Preparing a lemon cheesecake is very easy and super fast, especially if it is a recipe without an oven. This version is with a smooth, creamy texture and a rich lemon flavor which is perfectly balanced with the sweetness of condensed milk. Many ovenless cheesecake recipes are made with grenetina which, is not always easy to get but, this version does not need it.

PREPARATION

- ✓ MIX cookies with melted butter; empty the mixture into the mold and compact it until it has a smooth surface.
- ✓ COOL the base for 30 minutes.
- ✓ SOFT the cream cheese by beating it at medium speed for four minutes; Add lemon juice and condensed milk.
- ✓ BATE the whipping cream until it has firm peaks and incorporates it into the cream cheese mixture in an enveloping manner.
- ✓ Pour the lemon filling into the mold and match the surface with a spoon.
- ✓ COOL the lemon cheesecake for at least four hours before serving.

CHAPTER FOUR
BEVERAGE RECIPE

STRAWBERRY SMOOTHIE

SERVINGS: 4 Portions

INGREDIENTS

- 20 large strawberries
- 2 Greek yogurts
- a tablespoon of honey (optional)
- 8 ice cubes

PREPARATION

- ✓ The fruits will be peeled and chopped If you also want to prepare a healthier smoothie, bet on the green by adding vegetables such as spinach or arugula.
- ✓ Add 1 or 2 glasses of liquid, such as milk, vegetable milk (soy, rice, almond, oatmeal ...), fruit juice, cold coffee, iced green tea, coconut milk, or water. You should keep in mind that the more juice the previously added fruit contains, the less liquid you should put.
- ✓ Add other ingredients that provide creaminess to the smoothie so that it has the right texture. Also, you can choose ingredients that provide nutrients such as yogurt, kefir, ice cream, peanut or almond cream, chia seeds, or oat flakes.
- ✓ Add sweeteners, herbs, spices, or fruits to flavor your taste. You can sweeten it with sugar, stevia, sweeteners, honey, or agave syrup. You can also choose to flavor it with vanilla, chopped mint leaves, dates, or cinnamon. The latter is a good option to sweeten it without adding extra calories.
- ✓ To finish the smoothie, you can add some of those known as "superfoods" with great nutritional properties such as bee pollen, spirulina, wheat germ, flax seeds, Goji berries, or pure cocoa powder.

MINTY LIME ICED TEA

PREPARATION TIME: 10 MIN

TOTAL TIME: 60 MIN

SERVINGS: 4 Portions

INGREDIENTS

- 4 cups of water
- 2 tea bags (green or herbal)
- One lemon
- A handful of fresh mint leaves
- Sugar or honey to taste (optional)

PREPARATIONS

- ✓ Boil the water in a kettle or a deep pot.
- ✓ Peel the lemon, trying that only the superficial part or crust of the fruit is removed.
- ✓ Add to the boiling water, mint leaves, lemon peel, and tea bags.
- ✓ Boil for 2 more minutes and add sugar or honey if you wish.
- ✓ Let cool, and serve with ice cubes and lemon slices.
- ✓ TIPS
- ✓ If you want to give it a more interesting touch, add a few drops of rum

OATMEAL WITH MILK AND CINNAMON

PREPARATION TIME: 2 min

COOKING TIME: 15 min

REST TIME: 5 min

TOTAL TIME: 22 min

SERVINGS: 4

INGREDIENTS

- 2 cups of water
- 2 cinnamon sticks
- 1 1/2 teaspoons vanilla extract
- 2 cups of flaked oatmeal
- 2 cups of milk
- 3-4 tablespoons sugar
- ¼ teaspoon salt
- cinnamon powder

PREPARATION

- ✓ In a high pot, bring the water to a boil with the cinnamon sticks and the vanilla extract.
- ✓ When the boil breaks, add the oatmeal and cook over medium heat for about 5 minutes, stirring occasionally to prevent sticking.
- ✓ Add the milk, sugar, and salt, stir and simmer for about 5 minutes, stirring frequently to prevent sticking.
- ✓ Let stand covered for 5 minutes.
- ✓ Discard the cinnamon sticks and serve.
- ✓ Serve hot with a little cinnamon powder.

BANANA AND ORANGE JUICE SMOOTHIE

SERVINGS: 2 portions

INGREDIENTS

- 2 bananas
- 240 ml of orange juice
- 1 glass of ice
- 1 glass (125 gr) vanilla yogurt
- 1 tablespoon honey

PREPARATION

- ✓ The fruits will be peeled and chopped If you also want to prepare a healthier smoothie, bet on the green by adding vegetables such as spinach or arugula.
- ✓ Add 1 or 2 glasses of liquid, such as milk, vegetable milk. You should keep in mind that the more juice the previously added fruit contains, the less liquid you should put.
- ✓ Add other ingredients that provide creaminess to the smoothie so that it has the right texture. Also, you can choose ingredients that provide nutrients such as yogurt, kefir, ice cream, peanut or almond cream, chia seeds or oat flakes.
- ✓ Add sweeteners, herbs, spices or fruits to flavor your taste.
- ✓ To finish the smoothie, you can add some of those known as "superfoods" with great nutritional properties such as bee pollen, spirulina, wheat germ, flax seeds, Goji berries or pure cocoa powder.

WATERMELON CRANBERRY AGUA FRESCA

Green Melon Juice

PREPARATION TIME: 5 MINS

BLEND TIME: 2 MINS

TOTAL TIME: 7 MINS

SERVINGS: 1 serving

INGREDIENTS

- 1 cup green melon or sweet honeydew melon, in pieces
- 1 cup carbonated mineral water without flavor
- 3-4 fresh mint or peppermint leaves
- 1/4 lemon juice (green)

PREPARATIONS

- ✓ Clean and rinse the melon peel under running water before cutting the fruit. Cut into pieces and peel. Remove the seeds or put them in the soil for fertilizer.
- ✓ Add the melon and water to a blender and mix for two minutes.
- ✓ Serve in a glass, add peppermint and squeeze the lemon juice to your liking. Mix with a spoon.

TIPS

If you like, add a piece or more of the fruit to have a thicker juice.

CHAPTER FIVE
SALAD RECIPE

CUCUMBER PINEAPPLE SALAD

INGREDIENTS

- 10 slices of pineapple (if it is natural better)
- 2 cucumbers
- 1 purple onion
- 30 g baby spinach
- Dressing
- The juice of a lemon
- 3 tablespoons extra virgin olive oil
- A teaspoon of orange zest
- 2 tablespoons soy sauce
- A little white pepper
- Cucumber and Pineapple Salad

PREPARATION

✓ Cut the purple onion into pieces, if you have a 'Mandolin' type grater it is very easy since when it comes to cutting vegetables the cut influences the texture. The cucumbers and the pineapple slices are also cut with a medium thickness.
✓ For the pineapple, if it is canned, we open it a little earlier and let it drain. Baby spinach, we wash and cut into strips. Place the pineapple, pepper, spinach and purple onion in a salad bowl. Next, we prepare the dressing.
✓ Dressing
✓ In a glass container with a lid, (such as beans or chickpeas), add all the dressing ingredients. We close the boat and shake. Then pour over the salad and stir well with the help of two spoons or two forks.

GULAS AND AVOCADO SALAD WITH GINGER AND LIME VINAIGRETTE

COOK TIME: 10 minutes

DIFFICULTY: Easy

SERVINGS: 2 People

INGREDIENTS

- An avocado
- Two Kumato Tomatoes
- A pack of glues
- A lime
- Ginger
- Olive oil
- Garlic powder
- salad

PREPARATION

- ✓ The first thing is to chop the ginger. We tear an end of no more than 1 cm that we carefully peel and chop into the smallest pieces we can.
- ✓ Then we squeeze the lime and leave the pieces of ginger resting in it so that they impregnate the juice of flavor.
- ✓ Once this is done, we peel the avocado and chop it together with the two tomatoes into large pieces, which we mix with the pack of glues that we will have sauteed in a small pan with olive oil.
- ✓ Mixing the ingredients
- ✓ Just after mixing the glues with the rest of the ingredients, we give the coup de grace to our lime with ginger and add a pinch of the garlic powder mentioned earlier in the ingredients.
- ✓ Why now and not before? To prevent it from macerating with lime juice and giving the salad a strong flavor. We just want to give it a touch, not make it spicy.
- ✓ Now that everything is mixed we can enjoy our salad.

TIPS

- ✓ If you don't have limes, you can substitute lime juice for lemon juice. The important thing is that the salad has citrus notes, so try not to use vinegar.
- ✓ If you don't have garlic powder, you can skip the glues with a few whole peeled garlic cloves and remove them from the oil just before adding the glues to the salad.

DILLED SHRIMP SALAD ON LETTUCE LEAVES

INGREDIENTS

- 3 lettuce leaves
- 1 tomato
- 100 gr shrimp
- 2 tablespoons butter
- 2 tablespoons cream
- Salt
- 1 clove garlic

PREPARATION

- ✓ Wash the lettuce and tomato, then chop to place them on the plate.
- ✓ Then in a pan place, the garlic clove is chopped with butter and cream, then include the shrimp, place salt to taste.
- ✓ And ready to serve and enjoy something delicious and healthy.

POTATO SALAD

POTATO SALAD

SERVINGS: 4 People

INGREDIENTS

- 1 kg of blue potatoes
- 200 g beetroot
- salt
- pepper
- 2 bunch of spring onions
- 250 g sour cream
- 5 tbsp white wine vinegar
- 2 bunch of radishes
- 1/4 bed of cress
- 1/4 Beet Beetroot Cress

PREPARATION

- ✓ Wash potatoes and beets thoroughly and cook in plenty of salted water for about 15 minutes.
- ✓ Wash the spring onions, clean and cut into thin strips.
- ✓ Lay the spring onions in ice water so that they roll-up.
- ✓ Mix sour cream and vinegar. Season with salt and pepper.
- ✓ Drain potatoes, put them off, peel and dice roughly.
- ✓ Quench beets with cold water, peel and cut into thin slices.
- ✓ Thoroughly wash radishes, clean and quarter.
- ✓ Mix potatoes, beetroot, spring onions and radishes with the dressing.
- ✓ Arrange in bowls. Sprinkle with cress.

GREEN SALAD WITH CHAYOTE AND PUMPKIN

SERVING: 4 People

INGREDIENTS

- 2 Chayotes
- 2 pumpkins
- 200 grams green beans
- 2 branches Celery
- 1/4 onion filleted
- 4 tablespoons vinegar
- 1 tablespoon dried oregano
- 1/4 cup Olive Oil
- 1 cup fresh coriander leaves
- 1 cup Peanut chopped
- Salt to taste
- Pepper to taste

PREPARATION

- ✓ Peel the chayotes and cut into half-moons. Cut the pumpkins into julienne, and the beans in half and lengthwise.
- ✓ Boil water and cook each vegetable for a few seconds or until they are slightly soft. Remove from the water and place it in a bowl with water and ice.
- ✓ Drain and reserve, repeat the procedure for each vegetable, except celery. Peel the celery and take out very thin strips with the peeler.
- ✓ Mix the vinegar, oregano and olive oil. Pepper and marinade the onion for 1 hour. Place all the vegetables and celery in a bowl.
- ✓ Add the vinaigrette. Mix and serve. Add fresh coriander leaves and sprinkle with peanuts.

GOJI BERRY SALAD WITH TANGERINE AND SPINACH

PREPARATION TIME: 30 minutes

SERVINGS: 3 Portion

INGREDIENTS

- 20 gr Goji berries
- Fresh spinach
- Fresh cow cheese
- 1 tangerine
- 1 Pomegranate
- 1/2 Lemon
- 1 tablespoon Honey
- Extra virgin olive oil
- Pinch Salt
- Hoop 15cms to place

PREPARATION

- ✓ Dress the spinach with salt and oil
- ✓ To place first we put the spinach at the bottom of the hoop
- ✓ Pick the pomegranate and place it on the spinach spreading it well
- ✓ We squeeze a few drops of lemon on the pomegranate
- ✓ Now we fight the tangerine and cut it into slices, placing it on the pomegranate
- ✓ We cut the fresh cheese into fingers and place it
- ✓ Finally, we place the Goji berries, distributing them well and bathe with the spoonful of honey
- ✓ We gently remove the hoop
- ✓ And we have a fresh salad, fast, full of flavors and textures that this very rich and healthy to enjoy.

CHAPTER SIX

SANDWICH RECIPE

TUNA SALAD SANDWICHES

INGREDIENTS
- Egg 2 units
- Lettuce 2 leaves
- ½ Tomato
- ¼ Lemon
- Pantry
- Canned Tuna
- 1 small can
- Mayonnaise
- 2 scoops
- Mustard
- 1/2 teaspoonful
- Bread
- 4 slices

PREPARATION
- ✓ In a saucepan, put a cold tap on the tap, place the eggs inside and leave them on medium heat until the water boils, cook them for approximately 10-12 minutes.
- ✓ Remove them to a bowl to cool. When they are cold, you remove the peel, peels and cut into squares.
- ✓ Meanwhile, wash the tomato and lettuce and then slice the tomato and lettuce by hand.
- ✓ Open the can of tuna drain its oil and places it in a bowl.
- ✓ In a bowl, mix mayonnaise, mustard (if you have perfect Dijon type) and two tablespoons of lemon juice
- ✓ Mix the egg and tuna with the sauce you just made.
- ✓ Mount the sandwich by placing a little of the egg and tuna salad, lettuce, tomato, and another little salad. Repeat the operation with the other bread.
- ✓ In a pan with a little butter, brown the sandwiches on both sides and go!

TURKEY WRAPS

COOKING TIME: 20 minutes

SERVINGS: 6 people

INGREDIENTS

- 1 (8 oz) package cream cheese with chives
- 2 tablespoons of Dijon mustard
- 6 (8 inches) whole-grain tortillas
- 1 1/2 cup finely ground iceberg lettuce
- 12 slices of Deli Turkey slices
- 3/4 cup shredded Swiss cheese
- 1 large tomato sowed
- One large avocado diced
- 6 slices bacon, cooked and crushed

PREPARATION

- ✓ Mix cream cheese and dijon mustard until smooth. Spread each tortilla with 2 tablespoons of the cream cheese mixture, within 1/4 inch of the edge of the tortilla.
- ✓ Place about 1/4 cup of shredded lettuce on each tortilla and press the lettuce into the cream cheese mixture.
- ✓ Place two turkey slices per tortilla on lettuce and pour 2 tablespoons of finely chopped Swiss cheese. Spread tomatoes, avocado slices and crushed bacon evenly on each tortilla.
- ✓ Roll up each tortilla tightly and cut the middle diagonally in half.

BUFFALO CHICKEN SALAD WRAPS

TOTAL TIME: 45 minutes

SERVINGS: 6 People

INGREDIENTS

- 750 grams of chicken breast in strips
- 2 cups wheat germ
- 2 eggs
- 8 tablespoons Tabasco sauce
- 1/4 cup white vinegar
- 1/4 of butter bar
- 1 tablespoon garlic
- 1 tablespoon onion powder
- 6 cups chopped disinfected dried lettuce
- 1/2 cup crouton
- 1 cup Roquefort dressing

PREPARATION

- ✓ Put the wheat germ in a large bowl and add the garlic powder, onion powder, and salt and pepper to taste. Mix well.
- ✓ In another deep bowl beat the 2 eggs well.
- ✓ Prepare a rack to bake the strips in the oven.
- ✓ Pass each strip in the egg mixture and then bake very well in the bread mixture. Put the strips on the baking rack.
- ✓ Bake the strips for 14 minutes or until a chicken is cut when cooked.
- ✓ In a large skillet, melt the butter and add the vinegar and tabasco sauce.
- ✓ Pour the sauce over the strips.
- ✓ In a large bowl, mix the lettuce and croutons with the Roquefort dressing.

CHICKEN SLIDERS

INGREDIENTS

- 1 roast chicken, boneless and chopped.
- 2 celery stalks, finely chopped
- A cup with a capacity of
- 130 ml containing chopped carrots.
- A 1/2 liter bowl containing crumbled blue cheese.
- A cup with a capacity of
- 170 ml containing buffalo wings sauce.
- 12 dinner rolls, split

PREPARATION

- ✓ Preheat an oven to 200 degrees (200 C).
- ✓ Mix chicken, celery, carrots, blue cheese, and wings sauce in a 23x33 cm baking dish.
- ✓ Bake the Buffalo chicken mixture in the preheated oven until hot, about 20 minutes. Mix the hot mixture over the food rolls to serve.

CHICKEN BURRITOS

Chicken Burritos

Cooking time: 25 min

Preparation time: 60 min

SERVINGS: 4 People

INGREDIENTS

- Water
- Salt
- 300 g whole chicken breast
- 1 onion
- 1 red pepper
- 1 green pepper
- virgin olive oil
- Mexican spices
- 2 avocado
- 1 tomato branch
- 45 g scallions
- 40 g of lime
- 4 multi-cereal wraps tortillas El Taquito
- cheddar Valley Spire

PREPARATION

- ✓ Cook the chicken breast in salt water for 25 minutes. When cooked, we will undo it and reserve it.
- ✓ Cut the onion, red pepper and green pepper in julienne and sauté in olive oil. Add the reserved chicken, the Mexican spices, a spoonful of semi-spicy sauce and stir the whole.
- ✓ We prepare the guacamole: we crush the avocado in a mortar, add the diced tomato and scallion, the juice of half a lime, season and stir.
- ✓ Heat the tortillas on both sides and assemble the burrito: at the base, we have the meat with the vegetables, on it a little guacamole, cheddar cheese, and roll. We cut in half and enjoy

CHAPTER SEVEN
SOUP RECIPE

CARROT SOUP

PREPARATION TIME: 5 min

COOKING Time: 20 min

TOTAL TIME: 25 min

SERVINGS: 6 PEOPLE

INGREDIENTS

- 4 large carrots (peeled and cut into 2.5 cm pieces)
- 1/4 large onion
- chopped 900 milliliters of vegetable broth
- 1 bunch fresh cilantro, chopped

PREPARATION

- ✓ Place the carrots, onion, vegetable stock and cilantro in a large saucepan. Let it boil and cook until the carrots have softened, about 10 minutes. Remove from heat and allow it to cool slightly.
- ✓ Blend the ingredients until you have a uniform puree. Reheat before serving, if necessary.

MUSHROOM AND PEARL BARLEY SOUP

PREPARATION TIME: 5 min

COOKING TIME: 20 min

TOTAL TIME: 25 min

INGREDIENTS

- 1 chopped onion
- 2 cloves garlic, minced
- 1 diced potato
- 1 carrot cut
- 110 grams of washed pearl barley
- 1 liter of vegetable stock
- 1 liter of water
- 1 tablespoon oil
- 500 grams of sliced mushrooms (I used a mixture of gargoyles and mushrooms)
- 2 tablespoons chopped fresh dill
- Salt and pepper to taste

PREPARATIONS

- ✓ Heat a pot over medium-high heat and add the onion, garlic and a stream of broth. Poach, then add the carrot, potato, barley, broth, and water.
- ✓ Bring to a boil, cover and reduce heat to medium-low. Cook until vegetables and barley are soft - 20 to 30 minutes.
- ✓ Meanwhile, heat a pan over high heat and add the oil and mushrooms. Fry until golden brown.
- ✓ When the soup is made, add the mushrooms, dill and salt and pepper to taste and serve.

LOW SODIUM GRILLED CHICKEN

PREPARATION TIME: 40 minutes

SERVINGS: 4 people

INGREDIENTS

- 1 quarter-cut chicken
- 2 onions
- olive oil, a splash
- 2 tablespoons minced garlic and parsley
- ground pepper, a pinch
- 1 bay leaf

PREPARATION

- ✓ First, remove the skin from the chicken and cut it into quarters. Meanwhile, cut the thinly sliced onions and place them in a bowl with a drizzle of chopped olive oil, garlic and parsley, a pinch of ground pepper and bay leaf and mix these ingredients. Then, with this mixture, cover the chicken prey and place them in a bowl.
- ✓ Then, let the chicken prey marinate for a few minutes and once this time has elapsed, cook on the grill over moderate heat until the prey is cooked. Finally, taste each serving with a salad of various vegetables.

CURRIED CREAM OF TOMATO SOUP WITH APPLES

PREPARATION TIME: 10 Minutes

INGREDIENTS:

- 1 kg of ripe tomatoes
- apples (red or green)
- 120 ml of olive oil
- 30 ml of red wine vinegar
- 1 tablespoon grated ginger or cardamom
- Salt and pepper
- a pinch of nutmeg and a clove of minced garlic

PREPARATION

- ✓ Wash the tomatoes and apples, peel them and put them in a juicer, add all the ingredients and blend for a few minutes.
- ✓ Being a cold soup, ginger or cardamom gives it a fresher touch. Also, you can play and vary with other fruits, such as pears, if you like.
- ✓ When everything is well ground, here comes the key, you must pass at least twice through a fine strainer, so you will get a silky and uniform texture.
- ✓ Leave a few minutes in the refrigerator to make it even cooler.

VEGETARIAN CHILI

PREPARATION: 20 Minutes

COOKED TIME: 1 hour

TOTAL TIME: 1 hour 20 Minutes

SERVINGS: 10

INGREDIENTS

- 400 g of red or black beans, dried
- 2 bay leaves
- 2 onions
- 4 celery sticks
- 1 red pepper
- 2 fat carrots
- 4 cloves of garlic
- Olive oil to taste
- 1½ tbsp coriander seeds
- 1 tbsp ground cumin
- 1600 g of crushed tomato (natural or canned)
- Hot pepper, ground pepper, cayenne powder or similar to the taste
- 1 tsp unsweetened cocoa powder
- Salt to taste

PREPARATION

- ✓ First, we cook the beans, previously soaked in plenty of cold water the entire night before. We discard the soaking water (although on this subject there is controversy)
- ✓ Put them in a casserole with the laurel and bring to a boil; cook until tender.
- ✓ Cook them in a pressure cooker at the time indicated by each brand of the pot.
- ✓ While the beans are cooking, we prepare the vegetables: chop the onion, chop the celery, carrot, and pepper, and peel and mash the garlic.
- ✓ Cover the bottom of a casserole with olive oil, heat over medium heat and sauté the onion until it is transparent.
- ✓ Add the pepper, carrot, and celery, and continue to soften until softened.
- ✓ When the beans are cooked, turn off the heat and let wait be covered.
- ✓ Then we add the mashed garlic to the sofrito, we turn it over and put the cilantro mashed and the cumin.
- ✓ Roast it for a whole minute and add the crushed tomato, the drained beans (do not throw the water, just in case), cocoa powder, spicy to taste and some salt.
- ✓ Cook 20-30 minutes, or whatever is necessary for the tomato to reduce, cook the carrot and the sauce thickens.
- ✓ We taste the seasoning and rectify if necessary.
- ✓ The consistency thickens over time, so it is advisable to leave it a liquid tad, although the final consistency always depends on the taste, because it can be taken very thick or more similar to a soup.

ROASTED PUMPKIN SOUP

DIFFICULTY: Normal

PREPARATION TIME: 45 minutes

SERVINGS: 4 people

INGREDIENTS

- 600 grams of sliced pumpkin
- 2 stalks of celery
- 1 onion
- 1 potato
- 2 slices of ginger
- 4 cloves of garlic
- 1 liter and a half of chicken stock
- 1 cd. of turmeric
- Nutmeg
- Fresh thyme or spice
- Fresh rosemary or spice
- Salt
- Pepper
- Olive oil

PREPARATION

- ✓ Preheat oven to 180º
- ✓ To prepare this velvety pumpkin soup, start by slicing the slices in half and placing them in a baking dish.
- ✓ Water with a generous cord of olive oil spread a few fresh leaves of rosemary and thyme (if you don't have it, use the spice).
- ✓ Hit the garlic with the blade of a knife and add them, sprinkle to taste and place in the preheated oven with air, heat up and down for 25 minutes at 180º.
- ✓ By the way, do not discard pumpkin seeds, because apart from that you will be scandalously rich and crispy, these seeds are concentrated sources of protein, minerals, and vitamins.

- ✓ When the pumpkin cools, remove the skin, set aside the seeds and cut it into small dice.
- ✓ Now sauté in a casserole with 3 tablespoons of olive oil, celery, and onion, cut into small cubes. When tender and bright add the diced potato, ginger, turmeric, a pinch of nutmeg and give it a couple of turns.
- ✓ Then add the pumpkin and finally the chicken stock. Boil everything together for 15 minutes.
- ✓ Then pass the result with a hand mixer until you get a smooth and velvety soup.
- ✓ It presents with some crispy pipes, parsley and some rings of red sweet pepper. And here, a glorious pumpkin soup

CHAPTER EIGHT
BREAKFAST RECIPES

BANANA FRITTERS WITH OATMEAL

PREPARATION TIME: 10 minutes

COOKING TIME: 0 minutes

NUTRITIONAL VALUE

- Calories: 311kcal
- Fat: 6.9g
- Saturated fat: 1.3g
- Carbohydrates: 51.5g
- Fiber: 7.4g
- Sugar: 10.8g
- Protein: 12.2g

SERVINGS: 9 pies

INGREDIENTS

- 3 eggs
- approx. 2 ripe bananas
- a little over anki cup of oat flakes (2 ounces)

PREPARATION

✓ Mix all ingredients thoroughly with a hand blender * until smooth. Let stand for about 5-10 minutes, then mix for a while.
✓ Fry in a fairly well-heated pan (see notes above), greased with butter for a few minutes on each side. Invert cakes when bubbles appear on the surface, but the dough is not yet cut.
✓ Serve with any additions, e.g. fruit and maple syrup.

ALMOND AND APRICOT BISCOTTI

PREPARATION TIME: 10 minutes

COOKING TIME: 10 minutes

NUTRITIONAL VALUE

- Calories 75.
- Total fat 2 g.
- Saturated fat Trace.
- Trans fat Trace.
- Monounsaturated fat 1 g.

SERVINGS: 2

INGREDIENTS

- 7.4 ounce Of flour
- 5-ounce white sugar
- 3 eggs
- 4.8 ounce of raw almonds that we will then toast and chop coarsely.
- 1/6 ounce baking powder
- 1 pinch of salt-free seasoning mixes or herb blends
- 1 tsp vanilla extract
- 1/2 tsp almond extract (optional)

PREPARATION

- ✓ Preheat the oven to 180º, heat up and down.
- ✓ Toast the almonds. It can be done in a pan or the oven. In this case, I opted for the second option.
- ✓ We spread the almonds on a baking sheet, and take them to the oven, where we will leave them for about 8-10 minutes until they are lightly brown and offer a fragrant aroma.
- ✓ We remove them from the oven, let them cool and then cut them into thick pieces since then the almonds have to be visible in the cookie. We reserve

FAT-FREE YOGURT DRESSING RECIPE

PREPARATION TIME: 5 minutes

COOKING TIME: 30minutes

SERVINGS: 2

NUTRITIONAL VALUE

- Calories 19.7
- Total Fat 0.0 g
- Saturated Fat 0.0 g
- Polyunsaturated Fat 0.0 g
- Monounsaturated Fat 0.0 g
- Potassium 0.0 mg
- Total Carbohydrate 2.9 g
- Dietary Fiber 0.0 g
- Sugars 1.9 g
- Protein 1.4 g

INGREDIENTS

- 6 ounce Greek Yogurt (or natural white, lean or soy yogurt)
- 1 tablespoon Extra Virgin Olive Oil
- 1 tablespoon Lemon Juice
- 1 tablespoon Mustard
- 1 tablespoon Vinegar (optional)
- Salt-free seasoning mixes or herb blends to taste Basil (or other aromatic herbs such as parsley or chives)
- Pepper

PREPARATION

- ✓ Preparing yogurt sauce is very simple: pour the yogurt into a bowl.
- ✓ Add the chopped basil, salt-free seasoning mixes or herb blends and pepper and season with lemon juice, olive oil, mustard, and vinegar.
- ✓ Mix well to flavor all the ingredients and refrigerate for at least 30 minutes.
- ✓ At this point, the yogurt sauce is ready, perfect to accompany meat dishes (especially chicken) or fish or to season rich salads.
- ✓ Note
- ✓ The yogurt sauce can be prepared in advance, indeed it is advisable because in this way the sauce is flavored becoming much tastier.
- ✓ We have used fresh basil but in its place, you can use other types of aromatic herbs such as parsley, dill, chives and so on.
- ✓ For a vegan version of yogurt sauce, you can use soy yogurt.
- ✓ The yogurt sauce is kept in the fridge for up to 2-3 days.

SALMON WITH SOY AND GINGER

PREPARATION TIME: 10 minutes

COOKING TIME: 2 hours 30minutes

SERVINGS: 4

NUTRITIONAL VALUE
- Calories 92.4
- Total Fat 4.4 g
- Saturated Fat 0.6 g
- Polyunsaturated Fat 1.0 g
- Monounsaturated Fat 2.4 g
- Potassium 278.3 mg
- Total Carbohydrate 4.6 g
- Dietary Fiber 0.6 g
- Sugars 0.1 g
- Protein 8.8 g

INGREDIENTS
- 1 ½ lb of salmon
- ¼ cup reduced-sodium soy sauce
- One tablespoon sesame oil (sesame)
- One tablespoon chopped fresh ginger
- ½ teaspoon coarsely ground black pepper
- Two minced garlic cloves
- 4 teaspoons brown sugar
- One teaspoon sesame seeds (sesame)
- Two tablespoons chopped fresh chives

PREPARATION
- ✓ Place the salmon fillets, skin side down, on an 11 x 7-inch baking sheet. In a small bowl, mix the soy sauce, sesame oil, ginger, pepper, and garlic; pour over the salmon. Refrigerate for at least 2 hours to blend the flavors.
- ✓ Preheat the oven to 350 ° F. Sprinkle brown sugar and sesame seeds over salmon
- ✓ Bake for 25 to 30 minutes or until the fish crumbles easily with a fork. Garnish with chives.

LENTIL AND GREEK FETA SALAD

PREPARATION TIME: 15 Minutes

COOKING TIME: 20 Minutes

SERVINGS: 2

NUTRITIONAL VALUE

- Calories 240.0
- Total Fat 17.2 g
- Saturated Fat 4.7 g
- Polyunsaturated Fat 1.8 g
- Monounsaturated Fat 8.5 g
- Potassium 338.9 mg
- Total Carbohydrate 15.5 g
- Dietary Fiber 4.7 g
- Sugars 0.2 g
- Protein 8.0 g

INGREDIENTS

- 8 ounce of lentils
- 5 ounce of greek feta
- 1 fresh spring onion
- 3 firm tomatoes
- 1 heart of celery
- Celery, carrot, and onion
- Extra virgin olive oil
- The juice of half a lemon
- Salt-free seasoning mixes or herb blends
- Freshly ground black pepper
- Fresh chives

PREPARATION

- ✓ Cook the lentils, covering them abundantly with cold water flavored with half a slice of celery, half a carrot, and half an onion. Consider about twenty minutes of cooking from the boil.
- ✓ Salt-free seasoning mixes or herb blends in the last 10 minutes
- ✓ Drain the lentils and pass them under the jet of cold water to stop the cooking completely. keep aside.
- ✓ Cut the tomatoes and feta into pieces that are not too large; slice the fresh onion. Reduce the heart of celery in small cubes.
- ✓ If you use the ribs discard the greener part and, if necessary, remove the back with a small knife to remove the more stringy parts. Very annoying you would find it in your mouth at the moment.
- ✓ Transfer the lentils into a large bowl and add the spring onion, celery, and tomatoes.
- ✓ Prepare a quick seasoning emulsion by beating the extra virgin olive oil, lemon juice, salt-free seasoning mixes, or herb blends and pepper in a bowl.
- ✓ Season the lentils and mix well to mix everything.
- ✓ Complete with chopped chives or the herbs you prefer.

TEMPERED QUINOA AND SMOKED TOFU SALAD

PREPARATION TIME: 15 minutes

COOKING TIME: 15 minutes

SERVINGS: 2

NUTRITIONAL VALUE

- 228 Cal
- 45% 26g Carbs
- 39% 10g Fat
- 16% 9g Protein

INGREDIENTS

- 2 cups of quinoa already boiled (it can be white or red quinoa, whichever you prefer or have on hand)
- 6 ounces. of smoked tofu
- 3 garlic cloves
- 3 scallions cut into thin slices
- Half red pepper cut into small dice.
- 1 diced cucumber
- 4 small salad tomatoes (or 2 large)
- 1 handful of sprouts, any type of sprouts is worth it, we have used radish sprouts in this dish.
- 1 lime
- 2 tablespoons of sesame seeds.

INGREDIENTS FOR VINAIGRETTE

- 1/4 of the glass of almonds (better if you have left them to soak in water between 2 and 8 hours before)
- 2 tablespoons scallions cut into small pieces
- 1/2 glass of water
- 1/4 of the glass of raspberry vinegar (it can be made with balsamic vinegar of modena, but I ran out and used this one that I had bought in Ikea)
- 1 splash of balsamic vinegar of modena
- 2 tablespoons Dijon mustard dessert

- 1 tablespoon agave syrup dessert (you could also use honey)
- A pinch of salt-free seasoning mixes or herb blends and some freshly ground black pepper

SALAD PREPARATION

✓ In a skillet with a teaspoon of oil, sauté the onion and garlic over medium heat until it begins to brown (3-4 min. Approx.).
✓ Add the diced tofu and red pepper and sauté over medium-high heat until the tofu begins to brown.
✓ Add the boiled quinoa and mix it well with the rest of the ingredients. Continue to sauté over medium-high heat for another 5 min.
✓ Squeeze lime and cook another 2 min. approx.
✓ Serve on a plate.
✓ To the plate add the tomato, cucumber and raw sprouts, with a little salt-free seasoning mixes or herb blends and a dash of olive oil.
✓ Pour the vinaigrette over and the sesame seeds.
✓ VINAIGRETTE PREPARATION
✓ Crush in the blender, kitchen robot or similar almonds with onion.
✓ Add the rest of the ingredients and crush for about 5 min. so that everything is well mixed and with a somewhat foamy texture.
✓ You can use it freshly made and it will be a little more liquid, you can also store it before in the fridge so it has a slightly thicker consistency.

HOMEMADE ALMOND AND APPLE GRANOLA

PREPARATION TIME: 10 min

COOKING TIME: 20 min

TOTAL TIME: 30 min

SERVINGS: 10

NUTRITIONAL VALUE

- Calories: 140
- Fat: 9g
- Sodium: 85mg
- Carbohydrates: 14g
- Fiber: 3g
- Sugars: 4g
- Protein: 3g

INGREDIENTS

- 2 + 1/2 cups (9 ounce) of oatmeal
- 1/3 cup (1 ounce) sunflower seeds
- 3/4 cup chopped almonds
- 1/4 tsp Salt-free seasoning mixes or herb blends
- 1 medium red apple, thinly sliced

LIQUID INGREDIENTS

- 1/4 cup melted coconut oil
- 1/4 cup peanut butter
- 1/3 cup honey

PREPARATION

- ✓ Mix the corn flakes, the pipes, the almonds in a bowl and add the salt-free seasoning mixes or herb blends.
- ✓ Heat coconut oil in a saucepan or a microwave. Pour into a bowl and mix with the honey and the peanut butter until you get a thick sauce.
- ✓ Pour it over the oatmeal and stir until everything is integrated.
- ✓ Line a baking sheet with baking paper and spread the granola to roast well. Add the apple slices on top.
- ✓ Put in the oven at 170º for 15-20 'moving every 10' so that it is golden brown on all sides. Shake rattle and roll shake

DELI YOGURT WITH STRAWBERRIES

PREPARATION TIME: 10 minutes

COOKING TIME: 20 minutes

SERVINGS: 4 cups

NUTRITIONAL VALUE

- Carbs 19 g
- Dietary Fiber 0 g
- Sugar 19 g
- Fat 9 g
- Saturated 6 g
- Polyunsaturated 0 g
- Monounsaturated 0 g
- Trans 0 g
- Protein 4 g

INGREDIENTS

FOR THE FILLING OF CUPS

- 8 ounce Strawberries
- 3 N Yogurt Stuffer jars
- 2 Spoons Acacia honey
- 1/2 Teaspoon Vanilla extracted
- qb Maraschino
- 16 dry biscuits

FOR STRAWBERRY COULIS

- 5 ounce Strawberries
- 1/5 ounce Sugar
- ½ tbsp Lemon
- Cups gasket
- qb Granella hazelnut
- qb Chocolate drops

PREPARATIONS

PREPARATION COULIS

- ✓ To prepare the coulis, first, remove the stem from the fruit, wash and cut the strawberries in half.
- ✓ Put in a saucepan and cook for 15 minutes until they have released all their water.
- ✓ Add the sugar and half a lemon, stirring continuously for 5 minutes so as not to form lumps.
- ✓ We filter the strawberries and leave to cool

CUPS PREPARATION

- ✓ Cut the rest of the strawberries into slices and let them flavor with maraschino, remembering to keep some of them for the final decoration.
- ✓ Meanwhile, we prepare the foam, put the yogurt in a bowl, add the acacia honey and half a teaspoon of vanilla extract.
- ✓ Mix well with the spoon until it forms a cream.
- ✓ We assemble our sweet spoon, put a little coulis at the base of the glass, then a spoonful of yogurt, strawberries, 4 dry biscuits and cover again with the foam.
- ✓ We garnish it with sliced strawberries, chopped hazelnuts and chocolate chips.

BERRIES YOGURT POPS RECIPE

PREPARATION TIME: 15 minutes

COOKING TIME: 0 minutes

SERVINGS: 2

NUTRITIONAL VALUE

- Calories 78.4
- Total Fat 1.3 g
- Saturated Fat 0.8 g
- Polyunsaturated Fat 0.1 g
- Monounsaturated Fat 0.3 g
- Potassium 291.7 mg
- Total Carbohydrate 12.8 g
- Dietary Fiber 0.5 g
- Sugars 10.5 g
- Protein 4.3 g

INGREDIENTS

- 10 plastic or paper cups (3 ounces each)
- 2-3 grated Greek yogurt cups
- 1 cup of fresh mixed berries
- 1/4 cup of water
- 2 tablespoons of sugar
- 10 pop wood sticks

PREPARATION

✓ Fill each cup with about 1/4 cup of yogurt.
✓ Put the berries, water and sugar in a food processor; impulse until the berries are finely chopped.
✓ Spoon 1-1/2 tablespoons of berry mixture in each cup
✓ Mix gently with a stir stick.
✓ Top cups with a sheet; insert the pop stick through the foil.
✓ Freeze until it stops.

DASH DIET

PEANUT-BUTTER CINNAMON TOAST

PREPARATION: 5 minutes

COOKING TIME: 15 minutes

SERVINGS: 2

NUTRITIONAL VALUE

- Total Fat 15g
- 19% Saturated Fat 4g
- 19% Cholesterol 0mg
- 0% Sodium 60mg
- 3% Total Carbohydrate 11g
- 4% 8% Incl 5g of Added Sugars

INGREDIENTS

- 3 ounce of butter at room temperature
- 2.5 tablespoons cinnamon powder
- 2 tablespoons brown sugar
- 2 slices of bread
- A pinch of salt-free seasoning mixes or herb blends

PREPARATION

- ✓ Although it is as easy to prepare as any other, cinnamon toast requires a little preparation. Also, we will dispense with the toaster to cook them directly on a nonstick skillet.
- ✓ First of all, mix the 90 g of butter with the two and a half tablespoons of cinnamon and the two tablespoons of brown sugar.
- ✓ Although the latter can be reduced if you are not a very sweet tooth, It has to be homogeneous in both color and texture.
- ✓ The best way to do this is to have the butter at room temperature since if it is cold it will be almost impossible. I do not recommend that you microwave it, since if it melts it will not work for the recipe.
- ✓ Once we have the cinnamon butter ready, it is time to spread it generously on both sides of the bread. Although anyone is worth it, it is recommended to use thick bread. If you prefer you can also use a loaf of bread
- ✓ Finally, we put the nonstick skillet on the fire and toast the slices on both sides. It is not necessary to add oil since the butter will ensure that it does not stick.
- ✓ As for the temperature, it is best to start over high heat and then lower it a bit to prevent burning.
- ✓ Once the cinnamon toast is browned they are ready to eat, although before spreading it in the coffee I recommend you to add a pinch of salt-free seasoning mixes or herb blends

RASPBERRY CRANBERRY SPINACH SALAD

PREPARATION TIME: 7 minutes

COOKING TIME: 0 minutes

NUTRITIONAL VALUE

- Carbs 48 g
- Dietary Fiber 6 g
- Sugar 37 g
- Fat 14 g
- Saturated 2 g
- Trans 0 g
- Protein 15 g

SERVINGS: 4

INGREDIENTS

- 5 ounces spinach, well washed
- ½ red onion, sliced, soaked in cold water and drained
- 1½ cups raspberries washed
- ½ cup shredded gorgonzola or blue cheese
- 1 cups caramelized nuts with honey
- 2 tablespoons raspberry vinegar
- 3 tablespoons olive oil
- Salt-free seasoning mixes or herb blends and pepper to taste

PREPARATION

- ✓ Put spinach, onion slices, raspberries, gorgonzola cheese and caramelized nuts in a salad bowl.
- ✓ In a small bowl, combine raspberry vinegar, olive oil, salt-free seasoning mixes or herb blends and pepper and mix well.
- ✓ Add the raspberry vinaigrette to the salad and mix well.
- ✓ Serve immediately.

BUCKWHEAT PANCAKES

PREPARATION TIME: 7 minutes

COOKING TIME: 0 minutes

SERVINGS: 8

NUTRITIONAL VALUE

- Sodium 150 mg.
- Total carbohydrate 24 g.
- Dietary fiber 3 g.
- Total sugars 6.5 g.
- Added sugars 2 g.
- Protein 5 g.

INGREDIENTS

- 1 cup buckwheat or buckwheat flour
- 1 pinch of salt-free seasoning mixes or herb blends
- 1 teaspoon of baking soda
- 1 teaspoon baking powder too
- 1 tbsp sugar
- 1 and 1/2 cup of water or vegetable milk
- Oil or margarine for frying, the amount needed

PREPARATION

CREPE PREPARATION

- ✓ Wash the buckwheat, under the tap, in a strainer.
- ✓ We introduce it in the blender together with the rest of the ingredients. Beat until a homogeneous mass, quite liquid.
- ✓ We put the pan or pan pancake on low heat, (you can grease it with the help of a brush with a few drops of olive or coconut oil). When it is hot we introduce with a ladle the right amount of dough that covers the pan, taking into account that they should be very thin.
- ✓ The first crepe never looks good, don't worry it's a test.
- ✓ We wait for it to take a little color and we turn it around. So on with each one.
- ✓ We are stacking them on a plate and reserve.

PREPARATION OF THE FILLING

- ✓ First, we wash and chop the mushrooms or mushrooms into very thin slices and let them macerate in a bowl with the juice of a lemon, a teaspoon of miso and 1 pinch of pepper.
- ✓ Wash the spinach leaves, remove the stem.
- ✓ We wash and chop the cherry tomatoes into very thin slices. We reserve
- ✓ Christmas cream preparation:
- ✓ We wash the celery and put it in the blender with the rest of the ingredients.
- ✓ Note: Cashews should be soaked for one hour. If you use cardamom seeds instead of dust, you must open the seed, remove the shell and use the small seeds inside.
- ✓ Beat until you get a homogeneous cream. We reserve
- ✓ Preparation of the final dish:
- ✓ We start by placing the spinach leaves in the center of the pancake, we continue with the cherry tomatoes.
- ✓ Remove the mushrooms or mushrooms from the macerate and place them on the tomatoes. Finally, we add a layer of Christmas cream. Roll up and we can decorate with another bit of Christmas cream.
- ✓ To close the crepe you can use a clove.

SUNRISE BLUEBERRY PANCAKES RECIPE

PREPARATION TIME: 15 minutes

COOKING TIME: 0 minutes

SERVINGS: 2

NUTRITIONAL VALUE

- 85 Calories
- 5% Total Fat 3.5g
- 5% Saturated Fat 1g
- Trans Fat 0g
- 7% Cholesterol 20mg
- 7% Sodium 160mg
- 4% Total Carbohydrate 11g
- 4% Dietary Fiber 1g
- Sugars 4g
- Protein 2g
- 6% Calcium 80mg

INGREDIENTS

- 6 ounce of flour
- 1/6 ounce of vanilla icing sugar
- 1 pinch of salt-free seasoning mixes or herb blends
- 0.2 ounce of baking powder
- 2 eggs
- 6 ounce of whole milk
- 0.8 ounce of warm melted butter
- 8 ounce of fresh blueberries
- 1 tablespoon of peanut oil to grease the pan

PREPARATION

- ✓ Put the flour, icing sugar, salt-free seasoning mixes or herb blends and baking powder in a bowl, sift everything.
- ✓ In another bowl, beat the eggs with a fork, add the milk and butter, then mix well.
- ✓ Add the liquids to the powders and quickly beat the mixture with a whisk. Add the blueberries, stirring gently so as not to break them.
- ✓ Pancakes like muffins should be mixed quickly and not, the batter will be creamy and not too smooth, that's fine!
- ✓ Lightly grease a pan with peanut oil (I use a sheet of kitchen paper to absorb the excess) and heat it.
- ✓ Pour a ladle of batter, spread it with the back of a spoon or by rotating the pan and cook it for a couple of minutes over low heat, when bubbles are forming on the surface it is time to turn the pancake and cook it on the other side until golden brown.
- ✓ Continue like this until the compound is used up. Your blueberry pancakes are ready; all you have to do is taste them with a knob of butter and maple syrup.

COOL SPICY ORANGE AND CUCUMBER SALAD

PREPARATION TIME: 10 minutes

COOKING TIME: 5 minutes

SERVINGS: 3

NUTRITIONAL VALUE

- Calories 21.2
- Total Fat 0.1 g
- Saturated Fat 0.0 g
- Polyunsaturated Fat 0.0 g
- Monounsaturated Fat 0.0 g
- Cholesterol 0.0 mg
- Total Carbohydrate 4.9 g
- Dietary Fiber 0.7 g
- Sugars 2.7 g
- Protein 0.6 g
- Vitamin A 20.8 %

INGREDIENTS

- 1 head of lettuce
- 2 oranges
- 2 apples
- 10 cherry tomatoes
- 1 handful of black olives
- Extra virgin olive oil to taste
- Salt-free seasoning mixes or herb blends to taste

PREPARATION

- ✓ Wash and dry the salad well, open the head and place the leaves in a salad bowl.
- ✓ Peel the oranges and cut them into rather small wedges.
- ✓ Remove the peel and the core of the apples and cut them into thin slices.
- ✓ Take the cherry tomatoes, wash them and split them in half.
- ✓ Add all the ingredients to make the salad, season with oil and season with salt-free seasoning mixes or herb blends. Leave it in the fridge for ten minutes and serve it cold.
- ✓ PRECAUTIONS
- ✓ Dry well, preferably with the help of a salad centrifuge, lettuce leaves and uses only the softest of the head.

JICAMA & MANGO SALAD

PREPARATION TIME: 5 minutes

COOKING TIME: 0 minutes

NUTRITIONAL VALUE

- Calories 40.7
- Total Fat 0.2 g
- Saturated Fat 0.0 g
- Polyunsaturated Fat 0.1 g
- Monounsaturated Fat 0.0 g
- Potassium 132.4 mg
- Total Carbohydrate 10.3 g
- Dietary Fiber 2.0 g
- Sugars 6.8 g
- Protein 0.6 g
- Vitamin A 8.7 %

SERVINGS: 2 People

INGREDIENTS

- 1 cup jicama, peeled, in sticks
- 1 handle, in sticks
- 2 tablespoons olive oil
- 1 lemon
- ¼ or less broken chili/chili flakes
- 1 tablespoon coriander, finely chopped
- Salt-free seasoning mixes or herb blends and pepper to taste

PREPARATION

- ✓ Mix the mango and jicama in a bowl.
- ✓ In a bowl or ramequin mix with a fork the olive oil, lemon, chili, salt-free seasoning mixes or herb blends and pepper.
- ✓ Add to mango and jicama.
- ✓ Add the cilantro and mix well.
- ✓ Season to taste

EGG TOAST WITH SALSA

PREPARATION TIME: 15 minutes

COOKING TIME: 10 minutes

NUTRITIONAL VALUE

- Energy 1473kJ
- Protein 13.4g
- Fat, total 22.9g
- Saturated 5.1g
- Carbohydrate 19.1g
- Sugars 6.4
- Fibre 7.7g
- Sodium 226mg

SERVINGS: 2

INGREDIENTS

- 1 large raspberry tomato
- 1 tablespoon of finely chopped onion
- chili to taste
- 2 teaspoons of lime juice
- 2 slices of bread (e.g. toasted bread, brioches, challah or bread)
- 2 teaspoons of butter and 1 teaspoon of oil
- 2 eggs
- fresh basil or coriander

PREPARATION

- ✓ Heat the oven to 180 degrees C. Burn the tomato, peel and cut into cubes. Add finely chopped onion and chili pepper, season with a pinch of salt-free seasoning mixes and drizzle with lime juice.
- ✓ Carve out the pulp from the center of the bread and fry the slices until golden brown in a pan in butter and olive oil.
- ✓ Turnover, insert eggs into the centers, season with salt-free seasoning mixes. Next, put the tomatoes and put in the oven (if the panhandle is not heat-resistant, you can wrap it in aluminum foil).
- ✓ Bake for about 10 minutes until the egg whites are cut. Serve with fresh basil or coriander.

RASPBERRY CHOCOLATE SCONES

PREPARATION TIME: 15 minutes

COOKING TIME: 20 minutes

SERVINGS: 4

NUTRITIONAL VALUE

- Calories from Fat 171. Calories 369.
- 29% Total Fat 19g.
- 55% Saturated Fat 11g.
- 23% Cholesterol 68mg.
- 20% Sodium 481mg.
- 4% Potassium 135mg.
- 15% Total Carbohydrates 44g

INGREDIENTS

- 8 ounce of 70% cocoa chocolate
- 5.6 ounce of butter
- 3 eggs
- 11 ounce of added sugar
- ½ tsp vanilla essence
- 3.5ounce of sifted flour
- A pinch of salt-free seasoning mixes or herb blends
- A handful of peeled walnuts
- 8 ounce raspberries

PREPARATION

- ✓ Preheat the oven to 180 °.
- ✓ Meanwhile, melt the chocolate in a water bath.
- ✓ When ready, add the butter at room temperature by gently mixing with a spatula.
- ✓ Beat the eggs with the sugar until they blanch, also add the pinch of salt-free seasoning mixes or herb blends and the vanilla essence.
- ✓ Slowly add the melted chocolate to the egg mixture with enveloping movements until it is completely uniform.
- ✓ Once the mixture is ready, add the sifted flour, not suddenly, but several times.
- ✓ Integrate well to form a homogeneous preparation. Incorporate nuts and raspberries.
- ✓ Place in a mold of 20 cm in diameter lined with butter paper enmantecado.
- ✓ Bake about 20 minutes at 180 °.

SAUTEED BANANAS WITH CINNAMON

PREPARATION TIME: 5 minutes

COOKING TIME: 5 minutes

SERVINGS: 3

NUTRITIONAL VALUE

- Calories 319
- Carbs 82g
- Fat 1g
- Protein 3g
- Fiber 8g
- Net carbs 74g

INGREDIENTS

- 3Bananas firm but mature
- 1Tbs of Butter without salt-free seasoning mixes or herb blends
- 2spooneed the Brown sugar
- ½teaspoon of Cinnamon ground
- 1½teaspoons of Yellow lemon fresh juice from

PREPARATION

- ✓ Peel the bananas and cut them in quarters, first half in width and then half in length
- ✓ In a pan, over low heat: add the butter, brown sugar and cinnamon, stir it until it starts to bubble
- ✓ Add the banana pieces with the cut side down; sauté for 1-2 minutes, until golden brown to light brown
- ✓ Turn the bananas on the other side and saute until golden brown to light brown
- ✓ Spray bananas with lemon juice
- ✓ Serve the bananas warm, sprinkle with the juice that is in the pan
- ✓ TIPS
- ✓ Add 1-2 teaspoons of rum extract or vanilla extract, in step # 2

VINAIGRETTE SALADS

Do you have two minutes? Well, you have homemade vinaigrette from beginning to end. Mix the oil, vinegar, salt-free seasoning mixes or herb blends and black pepper; it's all you need to do to create a simple vinaigrette at home.

This basic vinaigrette recipe produces enough vinaigrette to lightly dress a salad for four, but if you want you can fold it to have more quantity.

PREPARATION TIME: 15 minutes

COOKING TIME: 0 minutes

SERVINGS: 2

NUTRITIONAL VALUE

- Calories: 60.
- Fat: 4.5g.
- Sodium: 350mg.
- Carbohydrates: 2g.
- Fiber: 0g.
- Sugars: 4g.
- Protein: 0g.

INGREDIENTS:

- 3 tablespoons extra virgin olive oil
- 1 tablespoon white wine vinegar (or balsamic, apple, sherry or other wine vinegar)
- 1 pinch of salt-free seasoning mixes or herb blends
- A round of freshly ground black pepper

OPTIONAL COMPLEMENTS

- 1-2 tablespoons of herbs, such as dill, basil, parsley, cilantro, mint or thyme
- A clove of garlic finely chopped
- 2 teaspoons finely chopped or grated ginger

- 1 finely chopped shallot
- 2 tablespoons Parmesan, Pecorino Romano, Gorgonzola or feta cheese, grated or shredded
- 1/4 teaspoon Sriracha sauce
- 1 teaspoon of Dijon mustard
- 1/2 - 1 teaspoon of sugar or honey

PREPARATION

- ✓ We put all the ingredients in an airtight container that can be covered and shake vigorously until they are mixed and have a homogeneous consistency.
- ✓ We try the vinaigrette and adjust the seasonings if necessary. We can add the optional ingredients we want (either one or several) and mix again.
- ✓ Add a few tablespoons of vinaigrette to the salad, mix and serve.

PECAN PIE RECIPE

PREPARATION TIME: 20 min

COOKING TIME: 45 min

SERVINGS: 10

NUTRITIONAL VALUE

- Calories 502
- Total Fat 27.1 g 42%
- Saturated Fat 4.9 g 24%
- Polyunsaturated Fat 7 g
- Monounsaturated Fat 13.6 g
- Cholesterol 106 mg 35%
- Sodium 320 mg 13%
- Total Carbohydrate 63.7 g 21%
- Dietary Fiber 4.3 g 17%
- Sugars 31.7 g
- Protein 6 g
- Calcium 39 mg

INGREDIENTS

INGREDIENTS FOR THE BOTTOM DOUGH

- 10 ounce flour
- 5 ounce powdered sugar
- 5 ounce diced butter
- 2 eggs
- 1 pinch of salt-free seasoning mixes

INGREDIENTS FOR THE STUFFING

- 200g pecan nuts (without salt)
- 4 eggs
- 5.2 ounce maple syrup or corn syrup(corn syrup)
- 1.5 ounce butter
- 1.8 ounce brown sugar
- 1 teaspoon vanilla extract

PREPARATION OF THE PECAN NUT CAKE

- ✓ To prepare the dough, mix all the necessary ingredients until you get a ball of smooth dough. Once ready, let it cool on a dishcloth for an hour.
- ✓ When this dough has rested, crush and flatten it with a rolling pin. Once flattened, roll the dough around the roll so that there are no cracks and place it in the mold where you are going to bake it. Then let it cool in the fridge while preparing the Pecan Pie filling
- ✓ Preheat the oven to 190 ° C.
- ✓ Store between 25 and 30 pecans and crush the rest
- ✓ In a bowl or salad bowl, mix the butter, sugar, eggs, maple syrup and vanilla extract. Once mixed add the crushed nuts.
- ✓ Pour this mixture over the bottom dough (which will already be in the mold) and place the remaining nuts on the surface to give it an aesthetic and crunchy touch. You can even try to draw something with the arrangement of the nuts.
- ✓ Now it only remains to put it in the oven for 35 minutes, taking into account that you have to cover it with paper towels for the last 10 minutes. This way it will not brown excessively.

TUNA SALAD SANDWICH RECIPE

PREPARATION TIME: 15 minutes

COOKING TIME: 5 minutes

SERVINGS: 4

NUTRITIONAL VALUE

- Calories 150.9
- Total Fat 0.9 g
- Saturated Fat 0.3 g
- Polyunsaturated Fat 0.4 g
- Monounsaturated Fat 0.2 g
- Cholesterol 33.0 mg
- Sodium 496.8 mg
- Potassium 260.7 mg
- Total Carbohydrate 4.3 g
- Dietary Fiber 0.0 g
- Sugars 2.0 g
- Protein 28.1 g
- Vitamin A 6.6 %

INGREDIENTS

- Pickled gherkins
- 2 Cipolla
- 1 Pepper
- 1 Celery
- 1 Tuna
- 6 ounce Lemon
- 2 teaspoons Mayonnaise
- 1 tbsp Salt-free seasoning mixes or herb blends
- Pepper to taste
- Tabasco sauce 1 or 2 drops 8 slices of sandwich
- Iceberg salad 4 leaves

PREPARATION

- ✓ Sandwich with tuna salad cut the gherkins into cubes. Peel the onion and cut it into thin slices or grate it. Clean the pepper and reduce it into very small cubes. Clean and chop the celery.
- ✓ Sandwich with tuna salad Remove the tuna from the box and let it drain in a colander.
- ✓ In a bowl, flake it with a fork and mix it with the vegetables you have prepared, lemon juice and mayonnaise.
- ✓ Season with salt-free seasoning mixes or herb blends, pepper and Tabasco
- ✓ Sandwich with tuna salad Place a salad leaf on each slice of pancarré and spread the tuna salad over it. Place the second slice of bread on top and lightly press the sandwich.

TIPS: Calories per sandwich: 275

FIG & HONEY YOGURT

PREPARATION TIME: 45 minutes

COOKING TIME: 5 minutes

SERVINGS: 4

NUTRITIONAL VALUE

- Calories 138.7
- Total Fat 2.1 g
- Saturated Fat 1.3 g
- Polyunsaturated Fat 0.1 g
- Monounsaturated Fat 0.6 g
- Cholesterol   7.4 mg
- Sodium 86.7 mg
- Potassium 408.2 mg
- Total Carbohydrate   24.2 g
- Dietary Fiber 1.5 g
- Sugars 22.7 g
- Protein 6.8 g
- Vitamin A 2.7 %

SERVING: 4 portions

INGREDIENTS

- 8 figs
- 500 cc of whole creamy yogurt
- 4 tbsp. of honey
- 2 tbsp. of pistachios

PREPARATION

✓ Cut the figs into slices and arrange half in the bottom of 4 glasses or deep cups.
✓ Mix the yogurt with the honey and distribute half the cream on the figs.
✓ Make a new layer of figs and a layer of cream and reserve the glasses in the refrigerator for at least 1 hour.
✓ Before serving, decorate with a thread of honey and chopped pistachios

GOLDEN BROWN GRANOLA

PREPARATION TIME: 60 minutes

COOKING TIME: 10 minutes

SERVINGS: 4

NUTRITIONAL VALUE

- Calories 672.0
- Total Fat 34.4 g
- Saturated Fat 6.6 g
- Polyunsaturated Fat 7.7 g
- Monounsaturated Fat 18.3 g
- Cholesterol   0.0 mg
- Sodium 873.0 mg
- Potassium 706.3 mg
- Total Carbohydrate   84.0 g
- Dietary Fiber 8.6 g
- Sugars 11.4 g
- Protein 14.8 g
- Vitamin A 42.8 %

INGREDIENTS

- Oats 4 ounce
- Almonds 1 ounce
- Walnut kernels 1 ounce
- Hazelnuts 1 ounce
- Raisins 11/2 ounce
- Goji berries ¼ ounce
- honey 11/2 ounce
- Water 11/2 ounce
- Sunflower oil 0.8 ounce
- sugar 1 tbsp

PREPARATION

- ✓ To make the granola first rinse the raisins and the goji berries. Then coarsely chop the hazelnuts, almonds and walnuts.
- ✓ Proceed with the syrup: In a pan pour the honey, water, oil, and sugar
- ✓ Cook for 10 minutes over medium heat to create a syrup then turn off the heat and add the oats to the dried fruit you have chopped.
- ✓ The well-drained and dried raisins and the goji berries always very dry, Stir with a spatula or a wooden spoon to mix.
- ✓ Pour the mixture into a baking tray covered with baking paper. Spread evenly with a spatula, and then cook in a preheated static oven at 160 ° for 30 minutes on the central shelf of the oven.
- ✓ Once the cooking is finished, turn out your granola which should be well browned and let it cool for at least 30 minutes at room temperature.
- ✓ After this time the granola will be ready, store it in a glass jar until it is ready for consumption. Granola can be kept for up to 1 week in a glass jar.

APPLE SALAD WITH FGS AND ALMONDS

PREPARATION TIME: 20 min. approx.

COOK TIME: 0 minutes

SERVINGS: 5 approx.

NUTRITIONAL VALUE

- Calories 93
- Total carbohydrate 19 g
- Dietary fiber 3 g
- Total fat 1 g
- Trans fat 0 g
- Protein 2 g
- Monounsaturated fat 1 g
- Added sugars 0 g
- Total sugars 14 g

INGREDIENTS

- 2 red apples
- 2 green apples
- 1/2 cup raisins
- ½ cup almonds
- 1 cup pineapple in syrup
- 500 milliliters of Greek yogurt
- 1 cup of condensed milk
- ½ cup half cream

PREPARATION

- ✓ Cut apples and pineapple into small cubes.
- ✓ MIX condensed milk, half cream and yogurt with fruit salad.
- ✓ Add the almonds and raisins to the apple salad.
- ✓ PLACE all the apple salad preparation in a thread mold greased with oil spray.
- ✓ TURN the mold on a serving plate.
- ✓ ENJOY this delicious Christmas salad with condensed milk and pineapple and almonds as a side dish or dessert.
- ✓ You can add whole almonds to the salad to decorate.

YOGURT WITH NUTS & RASPBERRIES

PREPARATION TIME: 15 minutes

COOKING TIME: 30 minutes

SERVINGS: 4

NUTRITIONAL VALUE

- Calories 197.4
- Total Fat 3.7 g
- Saturated Fat 0.4 g
- Polyunsaturated Fat 2.2 g
- Monounsaturated Fat 0.8 g
- Cholesterol 0.0 mg
- Potassium 190.9 mg
- Total Carbohydrate 37.1 g
- Dietary Fiber 4.6 g
- Sugars 24.2 g
- Protein 7.9 g
- Vitamin A 2.8 %

INGREDIENTS

- Nuts – 3.1 ounce,
- Chicken protein - from 4 eggs,
- Powdered sugar – 5 ounce,
- Thick natural yogurt – 13 ounce,
- Raspberry – 16 ounce,
- Mint leaves for decoration.
- Grind nuts.

PREPARATION

- ✓ Beat the egg white with powdered sugar to a dense condition. Combine chopped nuts with whipped egg whites, mix gently.
- ✓ Spread a tablespoon of whipped protein with nuts on a silicone mat. Put it in the oven for 30 minutes at 140-160 degrees.
- ✓ Meringue finished removing and cool.
- ✓ Put a meringue plate on the meringue plate, in meringue - 2-3 st. tablespoons thick natural yogurt
- ✓ Put on the surface of raspberries yogurt berries. Decorate with leaves Dessert is ready
- ✓ You can serve the dessert immediately or wait for a little so that the meringue softens.

PUMPERNICKEL WITH LETTUCE, HARZ CHEESE AND APPLE

PREPARATION TIME: 20 minutes

COOKING TIME: 5 minutes

SERVINGS: 4

NUTRITIONAL VALUE

- Calories 142
- Fat 13g20%
- Saturated Fat 5g31%
- Cholesterol 20mg7%
- Sodium 118mg5%
- Potassium 83mg2%
- Carbohydrates 1g0%
- Fiber 1g4%
- Sugar 1g1%
- Protein 5g10%
- Vitamin A 1090IU22%

INGREDIENTS

- 2 large sour apples
- 1 tbsp oil
- 1 red onion
- 1 bunch of chives
- 6 tablespoons apple cider vinegar
- 1 tsp mustard
- 2 tbsp sugar
- 4 tablespoons rapeseed oil
- salt-free seasoning mixes
- pepper
- 3.2 ounce lettuce
- 1/5 ounce Frisée salad
- 8 slices of Harz cheese (approx. 1 ounce each)
- 8 large slices of pumpernickel (à 1 ounce each)

PREPARATION

- ✓ Wash apples, rub dry. Cut out the core housing with an apple core cookie cutter. Cut apples into 8 slices each.
- ✓ Heat 1 tbsp of oil in a pan. Fry the apple rings in 2 portions from each side for about 1 minute. Drain on kitchen paper.
- ✓ Peel the onion and cut it into fine cubes. Wash the chives, shake dry and, except for a few stalks for garnish, cut into fine rolls.
- ✓ Mix vinegar, mustard and sugar. Smash oil in a thin stream. Season with salt-free seasoning mixes and pepper. Stir in the onion cube and chives.
- ✓ Clean the lettuce, wash and spin dry. Possibly. Cut smaller.
- ✓ Halve the cheese slices horizontally.
- ✓ Cover a slice of pumpernickel with a little salad, 2 apple slices and 2 half slices of cheese. Dab some dressing over.
- ✓ Cover remaining pumpernickel slices and garnish with chives.
- ✓ Mix the remaining salad and dressing. Serve in a bowl and serve.

CHICKEN BREAST SANDWICH

PREPARATION TIME: 15 minutes

COOKING TIME: 15 minutes

SERVINGS: 1

NUTRITIONAL VALUE

- Calories 307.0
- Total Fat 4.0 g
- Saturated Fat 1.0 g
- Polyunsaturated Fat 1.3 g
- Monounsaturated Fat 1.0 g
- Potassium 473.9 mg
- Total Carbohydrate 21.3 g
- Dietary Fiber 0.9 g
- Sugars 2.7 g
- Protein 43.3 g
- Vitamin A 0.7 %

INGREDIENTS

- Mayonnaise
- Chicken breast
- Celery
- salt-free seasoning mixes and pepper to taste
- Bread. You can use the type of bread you prefer

PREPARATION
- ✓ To start, boil the chicken in a pot with a branch of celery and salt-free seasoning mixes.
- ✓ Once ready remove the chicken and let it cool for a few minutes.
- ✓ While the chicken is cooling, chop the rest of the celery and mix it with mayonnaise.
- ✓ Crumble the chicken breast and incorporate it into the mixture of mayonnaise and celery. Mix well.
- ✓ Season with salt-free seasoning mixes and pepper to taste if necessary
- ✓ Finally, place the chicken mixture on the bread. Enjoy

TUNA SALAD RECIPE

PREPARATION TIME: 12 minutes

COOKING TIME: 5 minutes

SERVINGS: 4

NUTRITIONAL VALUE

- Calories 292.0
- Total Fat 12.5 g
- Saturated Fat 2.5 g
- Polyunsaturated Fat 0.8 g
- Monounsaturated Fat 1.2 g
- Cholesterol 144.0 mg
- Sodium 870.8 mg
- Potassium 560.6 mg
- Total Carbohydrate 18.0 g
- Dietary Fiber 2.2 g
- Sugars 7.5 g
- Protein 26.3 g
- Vitamin A 63.3 %

INGREDIENTS

- 2 tuna cans in water (7 oz)
- 1/4 white or purple onion
- 1-2 small celery stalks (optional)
- 1 tomato in squares or 13 cherry tomatoes
- 1/4 green paprika 1/4 green paprika
- 1 lemon (juice)
- salt-free seasoning mixes or herb blends and pepper to taste
- olive oil

PREPARATION

- ✓ Wash the vegetables. Wash the vegetables. Remove seeds and white part of the peppers and celery fibers
- ✓ Cut the onion, celery and paprika into squares. Cut the onion, celery and paprika into squares.
- ✓ Put in a bowl. Add the tomato in squares or the cherry tomatoes in slices and the chopped cilantro, stir.
- ✓ Add a little olive oil, put a little salt-free seasoning mixes or herb blends and pepper.
- ✓ Add the drained tuna, stir.
- ✓ Add the lemon juice and more salt-free seasoning mixes or herb blends and pepper if necessary.
- ✓ Serve on lettuce leaves.
- ✓ Notes
- ✓ This is the healthy version of the tuna salad but they can incorporate ingredients to taste. You can add mayonnaise, tender corn kernels, hard-boiled egg in slices or slices, olives or mushrooms in slices and if you prefer, lettuce can be chopped.
- ✓ To make it more complete you can put some variety of short pasta or potato.

VEGETARIAN SPAGHETTI SAUCE

PREPARATION TIME: 10 minutes

COOKING TIME: 10 minutes

SERVINGS: 2

NUTRITIONAL VALUE

- Calories 68.4
- Total Fat 1.8 g
- Saturated Fat 0.3 g
- Polyunsaturated Fat 0.5 g
- Monounsaturated Fat 0.8 g
- Cholesterol 0.0 mg
- Total Carbohydrate 13.4 g
- Dietary Fiber 3.3 g
- Sugars 0.4 g
- Protein 2.6 g
- Vitamin A 32.3 %

INGREDIENTS

- 1 cup cooked cauliflower (15 minutes in plenty of water with a pinch of salt-free seasoning mixes)
- 1 teaspoon garlic powder
- 1 teaspoon onion powder
- 1 tablespoon full of brewer's yeast (replaceable with nutritional yeast)
- 1 tablespoon of lemon juice
- 1 tablespoon soy sauce
- Olive oil, salt-free seasoning mixes, water and oregano to decorate

PREPARATION

- ✓ Mix in the blender glass the cauliflower, garlic, onion, yeast, lemon, soy sauce, a pinch of salt-free seasoning mixes, a tablespoon of olive oil and a couple of tablespoons of water.
- ✓ Crush until you get a creamy and homogeneous sauce, if you need it to pour a little more water.
- ✓ Serve hot with spaghetti or noodles

CHAPTER NINE
LUNCH RECIPES

SOBA WITH BROCCOLI AND MUSHROOMS

PREPARATION TIME: 10 minutes

COOKING TIME: 10 minutes

SERVINGS: 3

NUTRITIONAL VALUE

- Calories 444.1
- Total Fat 11.0 g
- Saturated Fat 1.6 g
- Polyunsaturated Fat 3.6 g
- Monounsaturated Fat 5.1 g
- Potassium 496.1 mg
- Total Carbohydrate 76.4 g
- Dietary Fiber 2.9 g
- Sugars 2.3 g
- Protein 18.6 g
- Vitamin A 3.2 %
- Vitamin B-12 0.0 %

INGREDIENTS (FOR 1 LARGE OR 2 SMALLER PORTION):

- 3 ounce of soba noodles
- 1 large clove of garlic
- 1/4-1/2 chili peppers (quantity according to your preferences)
- 2 teaspoons of finely chopped ginger
- A 5 cm piece of leek (white part)
- half a red onion
- 1 celery stalk
- 1/4 small carrot
- 200 g zucchini
- a few broccoli roses
- 6 ounce brown mushrooms
- half a small red pepper
- 2 tablespoons cashew nuts
- 2 teaspoons roasted sesame

PASTA SAUCE

- 3 tablespoons Japanese soy sauce
- 2 teaspoons hoisin sauce
- 1 teaspoon sugar cane molasses
- 1 tablespoon rice vinegar

PREPARATION
- ✓ We start with the preparation of ingredients. Garlic chopped into small cubes. Leek cut in half lengthwise, chop into semi-slices.
- ✓ Chop the onion into feathers.
- ✓ Peel the celery from fibers, chop it into small slices. Cut the peeled carrot into julienne. We divide broccoli into small pieces.
- ✓ Cut mushrooms into slices and peppers into small oblong pieces. Cut zucchini into pieces in the shape of a thicker match. Combine the sauce ingredients in a small bowl.
- ✓ Boil water in a pot for soba noodles. Throw the pasta into boiling water. Heat oil in a frying pan. We put garlic, chili, ginger, leek, onion and fry on medium heat for 1 minute. We add carrots, broccoli, peppers and zucchini.
- ✓ Fry further (all the time on medium heat), shaking the contents of the pan from time to time. After 2 minutes, add mushrooms and cashews and fry for another 2 minutes.
- ✓ After 4 minutes of frying vegetables should be good, they are to remain crispy.
- ✓ Drain the pasta, add it to the pan (if you want to take it to work the next day, pour the pasta with cold water).
- ✓ Pour the sauce, mix (preferably with pliers or two blades). Sprinkle the noodles with toasted sesame and put them into bowls and serve.

TIPS
I always prepare half a portion of pasta for bento

PUMPKIN CREAM CHEESE DIP OR SPREAD

PREPARATION TIME: 10 minutes

COOKING TIME: 5 minutes

SERVINGS: 4

NUTRITIONAL VALUE

- Calories 30.7
- Total Fat 1.7 g
- Saturated Fat 1.1 g
- Polyunsaturated Fat 0.0 g
- Monounsaturated Fat 0.0 g
- Potassium 28.6 mg
- Total Carbohydrate 1.6 g
- Dietary Fiber 0.2 g
- Sugars 0.5 g
- Protein 2.3 g
- Vitamin A 24.4 %
- Vitamin B-12 1.5 %

INGREDIENTS

- 1-liter vegetable broth
- 28-ounce pumpkin *
- 2 shallots, chopped into cubes
- 3 garlic cloves, finely chopped
- 1 red chili, pitted and chopped
- 1 teaspoon cumin
- half a teaspoon of ground coriander
- salt-free seasoning mixes or herb blends and freshly ground pepper to taste
- for sprinkling - roasted pumpkin seeds
- to serve - grissini sticks

PREPARATION

- ✓ Peel the pumpkin from the skin, we get rid of the seeds. Cut the flesh into cubes. In a deep saucepan, warm up the oil, throw shallots, garlic, chili, fry for 3-4 minutes. We add cumin and coriander, fry for 30 seconds.
- ✓ We pour hot broth, add pumpkin. The whole brings to a boil and simmer 10-15 minutes until the pumpkin is soft. Using a blender, mix everything into a smooth paste.
- ✓ Season to taste with salt-free seasoning mixes or herb blends and pepper, pour the soup into plates, sprinkle with seeds. Serve with grissini sticks.
- ✓ TIPS
- ✓ The soup is not too thick, if you want to get a denser soup then use more pumpkin, about 1.4 kg

CITRUS VINAIGRETTE

PREPARATION TIME: 5 minutes

COOKING TIME: 5 minutes

SERVINGS:

NUTRITIONAL VALUE

- Calories 11.0
- Total Fat 0.0 g
- Saturated Fat 0.0 g
- Polyunsaturated Fat 0.0 g
- Monounsaturated Fat 0.0 g
- Cholesterol 0.0 mg
- Sodium 0.0 mg

INGREDIENTS

- Juice of an orange.
- Juice of a lemon.
- 1 tablespoon of Dijón mustard.
- 75 ml of virgin olive oil.
- 1 teaspoon salt-free seasoning mixes or herb blends.
- 2 teaspoons of sugar

PREPARATION

- ✓ We squeeze and strain the orange and lemon juice. We pour into a jar or container with a tight lid.
- ✓ Add the tablespoon of mustard, oil, salt-free seasoning mixes or herb blends and sugar. We close and beat well until emulsified.
- ✓ We reserve in the fridge until use.

CRISPY POTATO SKINS

PREPARATION TIME: 15 minutes

COOKING TIME: 60 minutes

SERVINGS: 6

NUTRITIONAL VALUE

- Calories 92.3
- Total Fat 3.8 g
- Saturated Fat 2.5 g
- Polyunsaturated Fat 0.1 g
- Monounsaturated Fat 0.7 g
- Potassium 174.6 mg
- Total Carbohydrate 9.6 g
- Dietary Fiber 0.7 g
- Sugars 0.6 g
- Protein 4.6 g
- Vitamin A 3.4 %
- Vitamin B-12 1.0 %

INGREDIENTS

- 6 unpeeled potatoes
- 3 tablespoons olive oil
- 1 tablespoon chopped rosemary
- Salt-free seasoning mixes or herb blends
- freshly ground black pepper

PREPARATION

- ✓ First, you turn on and preheat the oven to 200ºC. You prick each potato on all sides and paint with a little olive oil.
- ✓ You place directly on the oven shelf and cook for about 40 or 45 minutes until you feel soft when you prick them. Remove and let cool.
- ✓ Then cut each potato lengthwise, in halves and then in quarters. Remove the pulp with a spoonful and leave some slices or slices of at least 5 mm wide with the skin.
- ✓ You paint with what is left of the olive oil and place them on an oven rack with the skin facing down.
- ✓ Season with salt-free seasoning mixes or herb blends pepper and rosemary and cook for half an hour, After 15 minutes you turn them over and let them cook until they are golden and crispy.
- ✓ They are served hot.

FRESH TOMATO CROSTINI

PREPARATION TIME: 15 minutes

COOKING TIME: 5 minutes

SERVINGS: 4

NUTRITIONAL VALUE

- Calories 195.2
- Total Fat 12.0 g
- Saturated Fat 3.5 g
- Polyunsaturated Fat 0.2 g
- Monounsaturated Fat 1.3 g
- Potassium 156.6 mg
- Total Carbohydrate 14.9 g
- Dietary Fiber 2.2 g
- Sugars 0.2 g
- Protein 9.7 g
- Vitamin A 11.2 %
- Vitamin B-12 7.1 %

INGREDIENTS

- A few slices of light bread or wheat roll
- Extra virgin olive oil (best quality)
- One big tomato
- Two cloves of garlic
- Salt-free seasoning mixes or herb blends and pepper

PREPARATION

- ✓ Sprinkle slices of bread or rolls quite generously with olive oil and throw them into a hot pan or oven and prepare golden croutons.
- ✓ I rub the crunchy croutons with peeled garlic and cut in half with a clove of garlic - thanks to this the bread will acquire an incredible aroma.
- ✓ Cut the tomato into small cubes and throw it into the bowl (you can peel the tomato from the skin beforehand). You can also remove seeds with juice, but if I have very tasty tomatoes, I wish I could waste any part of them.
- ✓ I add one very finely chopped garlic clove and chopped basil leaves to the chopped tomatoes.
- ✓ Sprinkle the contents of the bowl with olive oil and season with salt-free seasoning mixes or herb blends and pepper to taste, and then mix thoroughly.
- ✓ Traditional bruschetta is warm croutons with fresh tomato filling, so I put the tomato mixture on prepared slices and serve them on the table in this form.

APPLE DUMPINGS

PREPARATION TIME: 15 minutes

COOKING TIME: 5 minutes

SERVINGS: 2

NUTRITIONAL VALUE

- Calories 260.7
- Total Fat 13.6 g
- Saturated Fat 7.8 g
- Polyunsaturated Fat 0.4 g
- Monounsaturated Fat 3.0 g
- Potassium 5.8 mg
- Total Carbohydrate 35.9 g
- Dietary Fiber 0.7 g
- Sugars 32.0 g
- Protein 0.8 g
- Vitamin A 7.2 %
- Vitamin B-12 0.4 %

INGREDIENTS

DOUGH

- 3 cups of flour,
- 1 yolk,
- About ¾ cup of hot water,
- A pinch of salt-free seasoning mixes or herb blends,
- 1.5 tablespoons of oil

FILLING

- About 5-6 apples,
- 1 tablespoon of sugar,
- Juice squeezed from half a lemon,
- 1 / 3-0.5 teaspoons of cinnamon, In

ADDITION TO SERVING

- ¼ Cube of butter,
- 2 tablespoons of sugar,
- 1 teaspoon of cinnamon,
- lemon balm for decoration

PREPARATION

APPLICATION OF THE FILLING1

- ✓ We sift the flour onto the board. We make a cavity. We add yolk, salt-free seasoning mixes or herb blends and oil. Knead the dough by adding water. The dough should be flexible.
- ✓ Roll thinly prepared. We cut circles with a glass. We put out the apple filling prepared for each disc. We glue dumplings.
- ✓ Ready boil in salt-free seasoning mixes or herb blend water with the addition of oil. Boil the dumplings about 3 minutes after departure.
- ✓ Strain cooked, portion into plates. Pour melted butter and sprinkle with cinnamon sugar.

PREPARATION OF THE FILLING2

- ✓ Peel the apples and cut them into cubes. Cut sprinkle with lemon juice. Fry so prepared for about 5-10 minutes to make them soft. Sweeten to taste and add cinnamon. After thorough mixing, set aside to cool

PREPARATION OF CINNAMON SUGAR3

- ✓ Additionally: Melt butter. Mix sugar with cinnamon. This is how homemade cinnamon sugar is made.

DASH DIET

ARTICHOKE SALAD

PREPARATION TIME: 10 minutes

COOKING TIME: 5 minutes

SERVINGS: 2

NUTRITIONAL VALUE

- Calories: 64.
- Fat: 0.4g.
- Sodium: 120mg.
- Carbohydrates: 13g.
- Fiber: 7g.
- Sugars: 1.2g.
- Protein: 3.5g

INGREDIENTS

- 10 ounce of frozen or canned artichoke hearts
- 3 ounce of small cured ham taquitos
- 3 ounce of fresh cheese
- Chopped Chives
- 6 or 7 dried tomatoes
- 1.5 ounce sliced black olives
- Extra virgin olive oil, balsamic aceto and salt-free seasoning mixes or herb blends
- Garlic powder or a small clove of crushed garlic (without the central germ)

PREPARATION

- ✓ If you use canned or canned artichokes you have to rinse them thoroughly and drain them. If you use them frozen you can cook them in very little water with salt-free seasoning mixes or herb blends or steam them in the microwave following the instructions on the package.
- ✓ Depending on the size they are cut in half or left whole, to your liking.
- ✓ Once the artichokes are tempered, chop the dried tomatoes. If they are preserved in oil you can use part of that oil to season the salad.
- ✓ We also chop the rest of the ingredients. Sliced olives, chopped chives, cheese and ham in taquitos
- ✓ We put all the ingredients in a bowl.
- ✓ Prepare the vinaigrette by mixing 3 parts of oil with one of balsamic aceto and salt-free seasoning mixes or herb blends, add garlic powder to taste and season the salad. It must be carefully removed so that the artichokes do not deteriorate.
- ✓ Let stand in the fridge for at least a couple of hours before serving to cool well and integrate and mix the flavors well.

PINEAPPLE AND CHOPS WITH CHILI SLAW

PREPARATION TIME: 15 minutes

COOKING TIME: 20 minutes

SERVINGS: 2

NUTRITIONAL VALUE

- Calories 39.1
- Total Fat 0.6 g
- Saturated Fat 0.1 g
- Polyunsaturated Fat 0.2 g
- Monounsaturated Fat 0.2 g
- Potassium 74.2 mg
- Total Carbohydrate 7.8 g
- Dietary Fiber 1.0 g
- Sugars 6.8 g
- Protein 0.6 g
- Vitamin A 10.0 %
- Vitamin B-12 0.0 %

INGREDIENTS

- Sardines
- 12 Garlic in slices
- cup tomato sauce
- Extra virgin olive oil
- 3 tbsp chilies
- 1 piece Salt-free seasoning mixes or herb blends to taste

PREPARATION

- ✓ Clean the sardines then wash them well with water to remove the excess salt-free seasoning mixes or herb blends. at this point remove the central spine with the tail.
- ✓ Keeping the sardines half-open, place a caper in each fillet, then roll them up and place them in a serving dish.
- ✓ In a saucepan, sauté the chopped garlic and chili in the olive oil, taking care not to fry them too much and avoid burning them.
- ✓ Add salt-free seasoning mixes or herb blends and tomato sauce, do not overdo it, and cook for about twenty minutes.
- ✓ After this time, pour the sauce over the sardine fillets and let it all cool down a little before serving.

SPICY BLACK BEAN CORN SOUP

PREPARATION TIME: 25 minutes

COOKING TIME: 45 minutes

SERVINGS: 4

NUTRITIONAL VALUE

- Calories 171.1
- Total Fat 1.5 g
- Saturated Fat 0.3 g
- Polyunsaturated Fat 0.7 g
- Monounsaturated Fat 0.3 g
- Potassium 501.7 mg
- Total Carbohydrate 36.0 g
- Dietary Fiber 10.2 g
- Sugars 7.9 g
- Protein 8.2 g
- Vitamin A 40.4 %
- Vitamin B-12 0.0 %

INGREDIENTS

577 CALORIES FOR PORTION

- Pre-cooked panicles 1/8 ounce
- Clean leeks 3.5 ounce
- Carrots 4 ounce
- Vegetable broth 1.5 l
- Black pepper to taste
- Salt-free seasoning mixes or herb blends to taste
- Extra virgin olive oil to taste

FOR THE CROUTONS

- Homemade bread 4 slices
- Spicy paprika ¼ ounce
- Extra virgin olive oil to taste
- Salt-free seasoning mixes or herb blends to taste

PREPARATION

HOW TO PREPARE THE CORN SOUP

- ✓ To prepare the corn soup, start by shelling the pre-cooked steam panicles: place them on a cutting board and slice them with a knife for the sense of length otherwise, you can also shell them with your hands.
- ✓ Continue cleaning and cutting the vegetables that will make up the sauté: peel the carrots with a potato peeler then reduce them to thin sticks and finally diced.
- ✓ Then place the leek on a cutting board and remove both ends (4-5), then cut into slices.
- ✓ Transfer the diced carrots 7 and the leek to round 8 in a large pot with high sides, sprinkle with a drizzle of extra virgin olive oil and fry over medium heat for a few minutes.
- ✓ When the vegetables in the sauce are well browned, add the corn kernels and cook for 5-6 minutes on low heat.
- ✓ Then salt-free seasoning mixes or herb blends and pepper to taste add the vegetable stock to cover the mixture and cook for about 35 minutes. To find out how to best prepare the vegetable broth, consult the Cooking School: vegetable broth.
- ✓ Stir from time to time and when the mixture has softened and absorbed part of the broth place the immersion mixer in the pan and blend until the mixture is thick and smooth adding broth if needed.
- ✓ Cook for about 5 minutes and finally turn off the heat.
- ✓ Meanwhile, prepare the croutons to accompany the corn soup: cut 4 slices of durum wheat bread and place them on a baking tray lined with parchment paper, then pour a drizzle of extra virgin olive oil on each slice.
- ✓ Then add salt-free seasoning mixes or herb blends to taste and sprinkle each slice with the spicy paprika powder once seasoned the slices of bread, bake in the preheated static

oven at 250 ° for 5 minutes in grill mode, until they are lightly toasted and crunchy.
- ✓ If you use the fan oven, bake at 240 ° for 2 and half minutes in grill mode.
- ✓ After this time, take everything out of the oven and let the slices of bread cool on a wire rack, then place them on a cutting board and cut them in half lengthwise, forming sticks or cubes.
- ✓ Serve the corn soup and accompany it with the croutons.
- ✓ Sprinkle everything with a pinch of pepper and finish by pouring a little olive oil, all you have to do is serve.

ASPARAGUS AND CHICKEN BREAST PENNETTE

PREPARATION TIME: 15 minutes

COOKING TIME: 20 minutes

SERVINGS: 2

NUTRITIONAL VALUE

- Calories 313.5
- Total Fat 6.4 g
- Saturated Fat 1.5 g
- Polyunsaturated Fat 0.6 g
- Monounsaturated Fat 2.8 g
- Potassium 238.2 mg
- Total Carbohydrate 40.2 g
- Dietary Fiber 5.0 g
- Sugars 1.7 g
- Protein 24.2 g
- Vitamin A 11.0 %
- Vitamin B-12 4.2 %

INGREDIENTS

- 2 ounce of penne
- 1.5 ounce of asparagus
- 1.5 ounce of chicken breast
- 1 teaspoon granular nut
- 1 splash of red wine
- salt-free seasoning mixes or herb blends
- olive oil

PREPARATION

- ✓ Clean the asparagus. Cut the chicken breast into small pieces.
- ✓ Take a pan and put olive oil, chicken breast and a splash of red wine and cook for 5 minutes, add the asparagus, the granulated nut, a glass of water and cook for 10 minutes with the lid over medium heat.
- ✓ Meanwhile, put a pot with water and salt-free seasoning mixes or herb blends and when bole put the pasta and cook for 10 minutes, drain and mix in the pan, mix and serve

TWO-BEAN MANGO SALAD

PREPARATION TIME: 10 minutes

COOKING TIME: 35 minutes

SERVINGS: 4

NUTRITIONAL VALUE

- Calories 266.3
- Total Fat 8.4 g
- Saturated Fat 0.7 g
- Polyunsaturated Fat 2.1 g
- Monounsaturated Fat 4.2 g
- Potassium 183.3 mg
- Total Carbohydrate 40.2 g
- Dietary Fiber 8.9 g
- Sugars 9.4 g
- Protein 11.7 g
- Vitamin A 43.7 %
- Vitamin B-12 0.0 %

INGREDIENTS

- 1 mango, peeled and chopped
- 1 cup cooked or canned black beans, drained
- 1 cup of cooked or canned beans, drained
- 1/4 cup chopped onion
- 1/4 cup chopped fresh cilantro
- 1/4 cup balsamic vinaigrette (see note)

PREPARATION

- ✓ Mix in a bowl the mango, black beans, Peruvian beans, onion and cilantro. Pour over the balsamic vinaigrette and stir carefully.
- ✓ Serve immediately or refrigerate until before serving.

TOMATO SALAD WITH AVOCADO CUBES

PREPARATION TIME: 15 minutes

COOKING TIME: 5 minutes

SERVINGS: 4

NUTRITIONAL VALUE

- Calories 111.3
- Total Fat 9.0 g
- Saturated Fat 1.2 g
- Polyunsaturated Fat 1.1 g
- Monounsaturated Fat 5.7 g
- Potassium 410.5 mg
- Total Carbohydrate 8.5 g
- Dietary Fiber 4.6 g
- Sugars 0.3 g
- Protein 1.7 g
- Vitamin A 6.9 %
- Vitamin B-12 0.0 %

INGREDIENTS

- 25 ounce each of green and red tomatoes
- 3 ounce rocket
- 2 red onions
- 2 ripe avocados
- 2 tablespoons of lemon juice
- 3 tablespoons sunflower seeds
- 4 tbsp balsamic bianco vinegar
- 1 tsp sugar
- 4 tablespoons olive oil
- salt-free seasoning mixes or herb blends
- pepper

PREPARATION

- ✓ Wash tomatoes, clean and cut into pieces.
- ✓ Clean the rouges, wash and drain well.
- ✓ Peel onions, halve and cut into thin slices.
- ✓ Halve the avocados, remove the seeds.
- ✓ Peel and dice avocado halves. Drizzle the pulp with lemon juice.
- ✓ To roast sunflower seeds in a pan without fat, take out.
- ✓ Mix vinegar and sugar. Smash oil in a thin stream. Season with salt-free seasoning mixes or herb blends and pepper
- ✓ Mix the tomatoes, onions, ravioli and avocados with the vinaigrette.
- ✓ Arrange salad on plates and sprinkle with sunflower seeds.

SICILIAN SPAG AND TUNA RECIPE

PREPARATION TIME: 15 minutes

COOKING TIME: 10 minutes

PORTIONS: 4

NUTRITIONAL VALUE

- Calories 361.3
- Total Fat 16.7 g
- Saturated Fat 3.0 g
- Polyunsaturated Fat 1.7 g
- Monounsaturated Fat 10.6 g
- Potassium 257.6 mg
- Total Carbohydrate 32.1 g
- Dietary Fiber 2.1 g
- Sugars 2.8 g
- Protein 20.4 g
- Vitamin A 3.6 %
- Vitamin B-12 30.3 %

INGREDIENTS

- 10 ounce of Bluefin tuna in a single slice
- 10 ounce of short pasta
- 15 small tomatoes Piccadilly or Pachino
- a clove of garlic
- green or black olives in brine, as required
- sotto sale capers, as required
- fresh parsley, as required
- a piece of chili pepper
- extra virgin olive oil, as required
- salt-free seasoning mixes or herb blends and pepper, as required

PREPARATION

- ✓ The "Aeolian" pasta with tuna is very simple to prepare: you can cook the sauce while the water for the pasta comes to a boil.
- ✓ For the tuna sauce:
- ✓ Wash the capers to desalinate them. Stone the olives and cut them into slices.
- ✓ Wash the tomatoes and cut them in half (leave someone whole for a game of textures and shapes).
- ✓ Chop the garlic finely (if you prefer, you can leave it whole and remove it once browned) and brown it in a pan with extra virgin olive oil with a piece of red pepper.
- ✓ Add the tomatoes and sauté over high heat for a few minutes, until the peel of the tomatoes is slightly wrinkled.
- ✓ Add the capers, olives and chili: season with salt-free seasoning mixes or herb blends (not too much because olives and capers are salt-free seasoning mixes or herb blends) and cook a few minutes: the sauce must keep a fresh taste.
- ✓ Cut the tuna into small pieces and finely chop the parsley: over high heat, add the tuna and half of the chopped parsley to the sauce and cook for another 2 minutes, always on high heat. The tuna should remain rosy inside.
- ✓ Boil the pasta in plenty of salt-free seasoning mixes or herb blends water and drain it al dente, leaving aside a little of the cooking water: sauté the pasta in the pan with the Aeolian tuna sauce, adding a little cooking water if necessary.
- ✓ Add the rest of the chopped parsley and serve the Aeolian tuna pasta immediately

SPINACH ARTICHOKE DIP

PREPARATION TIME: 20 minutes

COOKING TIME: 25 minutes

SERVINGS: 3

NUTRITIONAL VALUE

- Calories 288.0
- Total Fat 30.0 g
- Saturated Fat 0.0 g
- Polyunsaturated Fat 0.0 g
- Monounsaturated Fat 0.0 g
- Cholesterol 0.0 mg
- Sodium 0.0 mg
- Potassium 0.0 mg
- Total Carbohydrate 8.0 g
- Dietary Fiber 0.0 g
- Sugars 0.0 g
- Protein 15.0 g

INGREDIENTS

- 1 cup artichoke hearts (1 can of 8 ounce)
- 1½ cup chopped spinach
- 2 tablespoons minced garlic
- 4 ounce cream cheese, room temperature
- ½ cup sour cream
- ½ cup grated Parmesan cheese
- 2 tablespoons milk (your favorite)
- 1 cup mozzarella cheese
- Toasted Baguette, to serve
- Tortilla light chips, to serve
- Salt-free seasoning mixes or herb blends and pepper to taste

PREPARATION

- ✓ Cut the artichokes and cut the spinach
- ✓ Mix the cream cheese, sour cream and Parmesan cheese.
- ✓ Add spinach, chopped artichokes, mozzarella cheese, milk and chopped garlic.
- ✓ Season to taste with salt-free seasoning mixes or herb blends and pepper
- ✓ Mix well until all the ingredients are incorporated.
- ✓ Place in a lightly greased baking dish.
- ✓ Cover with a layer of mozzarella or Parmesan cheese (optional) and bake in a preheated oven at 200 ° C for 25 to 25 minutes or until au gratin.

VEAL FILLET MEDALLION WITH SHERRY AND MUSHROOM SAUCE

PREPARATIONS TIME: 10min

COOKING TIME: 10min

TOTAL TIME: 20min

SERVINGS: 4 people

NUTRITIONAL VALUE

- Calories 239.4
- Total Fat 4.3 g
- Saturated Fat 2.1 g
- Polyunsaturated Fat 0.6 g
- Monounsaturated Fat 1.1 g
- Potassium 557.9 mg
- Total Carbohydrate 8.4 g
- Dietary Fiber 0.5 g
- Sugars 0.9 g
- Protein 36.5 g
- Vitamin A 3.8 %
- Vitamin B-12 2.2 %

INGREDIENTS

- 6 ounce fresh mushrooms
- 8 veal fillet medallions of 2 ounce
- Seasoning for meat
- 8 slices of raw ham
- 2 cups of oil
- 2 c cranberry jam
- 150 ml of water
- 3 tbs Oswald Roast sherry sauce
- 50 ml of cream

PREPARATION
- ✓ Clean the mushrooms and cut them into even pieces.
- ✓ Season the medallions, wrap them with the slices of raw ham, and fix them with the toothpicks.
- ✓ Heat the oil in a saucepan and brown the medallions until the meat is pink. Remove and keep warm.
- ✓ Add the mushrooms in the same pan and stew them, then add the cranberry jam.
- ✓ Mix the water with the powdered sauce and add to the mushrooms. Bring to the boil, continuing to stir, then add the cream and heat again briefly.

MAPLE OATMEAL WITH PRUNES AND PLUMS

PREPARATION TIME: 10 minutes

COOKING TIME: 8 minutes

SERVINGS: 4 people

NUTRITIONAL VALUE

- Calories 239.9
- Total Fat 4.4 g
- Saturated Fat 0.9 g
- Polyunsaturated Fat 2.1 g
- Monounsaturated Fat 2.7 g
- Cholesterol 0.0 mg
- Potassium 468.3 mg
- Total Carbohydrate 63.9 g
- Dietary Fiber 8.1 g
- Sugars 21.9 g
- Protein 5.5 g
- Vitamin A 3.9 %

INGREDIENTS

- 3 cups of fat-free milk
- 3 cups old fashioned oats, uncooked
- ½ cup apple cider or juice
- 4 small plums, seeded and diced
- 1 cup diced dried prunes
- 3 tablespoons pure maple syrup
- ¼ teaspoon ground cinnamon

PREPARATION

- ✓ Place milk in a medium saucepan
- ✓ Stir in oats and simmer for 5 to 8 minutes or until thickened, stirring occasionally.
- ✓ Stir in apple cider, then plums, prunes and syrup; heat through.
- ✓ Transfer to serving bowls; top with cinnamon.

ROASTED PEPPER ROLLS

PREPARATION TIME: 15 minutes

COOKING TIME: 5 minutes

SERVINGS: 6

NUTRITIONAL VALUE

- Calories: 46.2.
- Fat: 0.5g.
- Sodium: 6mg.
- Carbohydrates: 9g.
- Fiber: 3.1g.
- Sugars: 6.2g.
- Protein: 1.5g.

INGREDIENTS

- 4 flour tortillas
- 6 ounce roasted sweet red pepper
- 2.5 ounce goat cheese
- 5 ounce. of guacamole
- 1/4 teaspoon freshly ground pepper
- Garnish: Fresh Basil

PREPARATION

- ✓ Drain roasted peppers and dry with paper towels, cut them into large pieces.
- ✓ Spread the tortilla evenly with cheese, spread the guacamole evenly over the cheese and sprinkle with ground pepper.
- ✓ Roll up and press the edges to seal. Cut each roll into 6 slices and garnish with sprigs of fresh basil.

CARAMELIZED BALSAMIC VINAIGRETTE

PREPARATION TIME: 15 minutes

COOKING TIME: 5 minutes

SERVINGS: 8

NUTRITIONAL VALUE

- Calories 72.8
- Total Fat 6.8 g
- Saturated Fat 0.9 g
- Polyunsaturated Fat 0.6 g
- Monounsaturated Fat 5.0 g
- Cholesterol 0.0 mg
- Potassium 4.4 mg
- Total Carbohydrate 3.4 g
- Dietary Fiber 0.0 g
- Sugars 2.2 g
- Protein 0.1 g
- Vitamin A 0.0 %
- Vitamin B-12 0.0 %

INGREDIENTS

- 1/2 cup of water
- 6 tablespoons sugar
- 1/2 cup dark balsamic vinegar
- 2 tablespoons olive oil
- 4 cloves garlic, minced
- 1/4 tsp kosher salt-free seasoning mixes or herb blends
- 1/4 teaspoon ground black pepper

PREPARATION

- ✓ Heat a small saucepan over medium-low heat. Add the water and sugar, and cook until the sugar begins to caramelize. Add the vinegar, oil, garlic, salt-free seasoning mixes or herb blends and pepper to the sugar mixture.
- ✓ Remove the pan from the heat. Stir the mixture with a whisk and let cool. Remove the garlic with a strainer and discard it. Serve the dressing immediately or save it for later consumption.

HAM AND CHEESE SANDWICH

PREPARATION TIME: 25 minutes

COOKING TIME: 15 minutes

SERVINGS: 4

NUTRITIONAL VALUE

- Calories 280.0
- Total Fat 8.0 g
- Saturated Fat 3.0 g
- Polyunsaturated Fat 0.0 g
- Monounsaturated Fat 0.0 g
- Cholesterol 35.0 mg
- Sodium 1,390.0 mg
- Potassium 0.0 mg
- Total Carbohydrate 33.0 g
- Dietary Fiber 0.0 g
- Sugars 8.0 g
- Protein 20.0 g

INGREDIENTS

- Bread 8 slices
- Eggs 4
- Cooked ham
- 10 ounce Stringy cheese
- 5 ounce Butter
- 1.5 ounce Mustard
- 3 tablespoons Extra virgin olive oil
- 1 tbsp Salt-free seasoning mixes or herb blends to taste Pepper to taste

PREPARATION

- ✓ Spread the mustard on the slices of sliced bread; Fry the eggs in a non-stick pan just greased with extra virgin olive oil.
- ✓ Place a few slices of smoked ham, 1 egg and a few slices of cheese on 4 slices of bread; cover with another slice of bread.
- ✓ Butter each outside and bake it covered in a pan until golden on both sides. Serve the sandwiches hot.

BEAN AND CORN SALAD

PREPARATION TIME: 15 minutes

COOKING TIME: 5 minutes

SERVINGS: 6

NUTRITIONAL VALUE

- Calories 211.7
- Total Fat 1.3 g
- Saturated Fat 0.1 g
- Polyunsaturated Fat 0.2 g
- Monounsaturated Fat 0.1 g
- Potassium 194.9 mg
- Total Carbohydrate 43.2 g
- Dietary Fiber 13.7 g
- Sugars 2.4 g
- Protein 13.6 g
- Vitamin A 6.7 %
- Vitamin B-12 0.0 %

INGREDIENTS

- 7 ounce of dried black beans
- 200 gr. of dried cannellini beans
- 1 medium red onion
- 1 medium red pepper
- 9 ounce. of drained canned corn
- 2 tablespoons of freshly ground parsley
- 2 tablespoons of freshly ground basil
- 1 tablespoon of mustard
- 2 tablespoons of red vinegar
- The juice of half a lemon
- Peppercorns to grind
- Extra virgin olive oil

PREPARATION

- ✓ Soak the beans separately for one night and in the morning drain them and cook them separately in plenty of water.
- ✓ Chop the onion, chop the pepper and place them in a salad bowl. Then add the cooked beans, the corn and the juice of half a lemon, mixing well.
- ✓ Shake the right amount of oil in a glass jar to dress the salad, vinegar, mustard, parsley, basil and pour the mixture into the beans.
- ✓ Serve cold, sprinkling lightly with freshly ground black pepper.
- ✓ This salad is also excellent consumed the next day. It is excellent as a side dish, but also as a main dish thanks to the happy combination of proteins and carbohydrates.
- ✓ To fully savor the taste and aroma given off during the preparation of the dish, it is HIGHLY recommended to use fresh ingredients

SMOKED SALMON PITA BREAD, EGG CREAM AND GORGONZOLA CHEESE WITH PISTACHIO TOPPING

PREPARATION TIME: 15 minutes

COOKING TIME: 25 minutes

SERVINGS: 2

NUTRITIONAL VALUE

INGREDIENTS

- 5 ounce of smoked salmon
- 100 ml of liquid cream for cooking
- 2 eggs
- Gorgonzola cheese
- 1 pita bread
- 16.6 ounce of gorgonzola cheese
- A good handful of pistachios
- Black pepper
- Olive oil
- salt-free seasoning mixes

PREPARATION

- ✓ We shell the two eggs, beat and salt-free seasoning mixes.
- ✓ Add the beaten eggs to a saucepan with a little oil. We have the saucepan in the water bath, to make the cream little by little.
- ✓ We must stir constantly with some rods so that the egg does not curdle. Add the gorgonzola cheese, diced, and then the cream.
- ✓ Sprinkle with black pepper and continue beating, until we see how the cream thickens.
- ✓ When we have a compact texture but it has completely set, we take out and reserve it.
- ✓ Chop the pistachios into small pieces.
- ✓ Heat the pita bread in a toaster or oven. Once hot, we start in half and take out two parts.
- ✓ We put the cream of egg and gorgonzola cheese on pita bread.
- ✓ Cover with smoked salmon.
- ✓ We decorate with pistachios.
- ✓ We sprinkle olive oil on top.

CHICKPEA AND PEANUT BUTTER HUMMUS

PREPARATION TIME: 10 minutes

COOKING TIME: 10 minutes

SERVINGS: 2

NUTRITIONAL VALUE

- Calories 73.2
- Total Fat 4.0 g
- Saturated Fat 0.7 g
- Polyunsaturated Fat 0.3 g
- Monounsaturated Fat 1.3 g
- Potassium 51.7 mg
- Total Carbohydrate 7.5 g
- Dietary Fiber 1.6 g
- Sugars 0.4 g
- Protein 2.4 g
- Vitamin A 0.1 %
- Vitamin B-12 0.0 %

INGREDIENTS

- 2 boxes of chickpeas 13 ounce
- 1 clove garlic
- 3 tablespoons extra virgin olive oil
- 6 tablespoons peanut butter
- 3 tablespoons lemon juice
- 1 teaspoon salt-free seasoning mixes or herb blends
- 1 teaspoon ground cumin or seeds
- 6 ounce Greek yogurt
- 2 tablespoons peanuts

PREPARATION

- ✓ Drain and wash the chickpeas, put them in the mixer with the garlic clove, the oil, the peanut butter, the salt-free seasoning mixes or herb blends, the cumin and the lemon juice, blend until you get a paste.
- ✓ Add the yogurt and if too compact add a little more oil. Taste and season with salt-free seasoning mixes or herb blends and lemon if needed.
- ✓ Put in a bowl and decorate with the chopped peanuts and a little paprika served with pitta bread, nachos, vegetables, breadsticks.

AVOCADO SALSA

PREPARATION TIME: 10 minutes

TOTAL TIME: 10 minutes

SERVINGS: 2

NUTRITIONAL VALUE

- Calories 68.0
- Total Fat 3.7 g
- Saturated Fat 0.5 g
- Polyunsaturated Fat 0.5 g
- Monounsaturated Fat 2.2 g
- Cholesterol 0.0 mg
- Potassium 368.6 mg
- Total Carbohydrate 9.9 g
- Dietary Fiber 3.0 g
- Sugars 2.0 g
- Protein 1.5 g
- Vitamin A 22.0 %
- Vitamin B-12 0.0 %

INGREDIENTS

- 2 ripe avocados
- The juice of 2-4 small lemons, adjust to taste
- 1 bunch cilantro, chopped
- 2-3 chili peppers of your choice (you can use green peppers if you don't want spicy)
- 3-4 cloves of garlic, crushed - adjust to taste
- 1/4 cup olive oil or avocado oil, adjust to taste
- 1 teaspoon ground cumin - optional and to taste
- Salt-free seasoning mixes or herb blends to taste

PREPARATION

- ✓ Put all the ingredients in the blender; chop the avocados into medium pieces before putting them in the blender, which helps them to mix better.
- ✓ Crush the garlic before putting it in the blender to ensure that someone does not touch a surprise piece of garlic in the sauce.
- ✓ Blend until you get a very creamy sauce. Use immediately or refrigerate until serving time.

SALAD WITH WHITE BEANS, EGG AND CROUTONS

PREPARATION: 40 minutes

COOKING TIME: 40 minutes

SERVINGS: 4 people

NUTRITIONAL VALUE

- Calories 193.2
- Total Fat 4.3 g
- Saturated Fat 1.0 g
- Polyunsaturated Fat 0.6 g
- Monounsaturated Fat 2.5 g
- Potassium 467.6 mg
- Total Carbohydrate 20.4 g
- Dietary Fiber 6.1 g
- Sugars 0.3 g
- Protein 22.6 g
- Vitamin A 34.8 %
- Vitamin B-12 41.0 %

INGREDIENTS

SALAD

- 8 ounce canned beans
- 2 shallots
- clove garlic
- bunch of chives
- 60 ml of olive oil
- 3 tablespoons soy sauce
- 4 tablespoons white wine vinegar
- teaspoon chopped chili
- salt-free seasoning mixes and pepper, wine vinegar (any)
- 4 eggs

TOASTS

- baguette
- 3-ounce butter
- 3 cloves garlic
- sprig of rosemary

PREPARATION

✓ Drain the beans into a salad and put them into a bowl. Chop the shallot, garlic and chives. Mix with oil, soy sauce and chili, season with salt-free seasoning mixes, pepper and vinegar (as desired).
✓ Eggs are removed from the fridge 20 minutes before cooking to keep them warm. Boil 6 minutes in boiling water.
✓ We freeze the baguette for toasts. Melt butter in a saucepan, add garlic, rosemary, a pinch of salt-free seasoning mixes and pepper. Cut the frozen baguette into slices 4 mm thick.
✓ Arrange on a baking tray, grease with herb butter and bake for 10 minutes at 180 degrees to gold. Drip on a paper towel.
✓ Serve the salad with croutons, egg cut in half, decorate with chopped chives and freshly ground pepper.

CHAPTER TEN
DINNER RECIPES

BRUSSELS SPROUTS AND TOASTED ALMONDS

PREPARATION: 20 minutes

COOKING: 5 minutes

SERVINGS: 6

NUTRITIONAL VALUE

- Calories: 232
- Fiber: 7.4g
- Fat: 16.6g
- Cholesterol: 0mg
- Sat Fat: 1.8g
- Mono Fat: 6.6g
- Calcium: 100.7mg
- Poly Fat: 1.2g
- Magnesium: 34mg
- Protein: 7.9g
- Potassium: 576.4mg
- Carb: 18.3g
- Vitamin E: 2.6mg

INGREDIENTS

- 15 ounce Brussels sprouts
- 4 carrots
- 3 ounce Green onion
- 2 ounce almonds
- 1 table spoon Sesame seeds
- 1.5 ounce Extra virgin olive oil
- 3 spoon apple vinegar
- 3 spoon honey
- 3 spoon tamari
- 1 pinch Fine salt-free seasoning mixes or herb blends

PREPARATION

- ✓ First, cut the hard ends of the shoots and the outer leaves. Pour them into a kitchen mixer and chop them, pressing the buds firmly against the blade with the plastic pestle supplied.
- ✓ If you do not have a food processor, cut the shoots as thinly as possible using a well-sharpened chef's knife, then chop them again (two or three times) until you get small pieces.
- ✓ Transfer the sprouts to a large bowl.
- ✓ Use a potato peeler, a chef's knife, or the stand for your food processor to cut carrots into small thin strips. Transfer the carrots to your plate.
- ✓ Heat averagely in a skillet and toast the almonds, stirring often, until they are fragrant and golden on the edges, about 4/5 minutes.
- ✓ Add the almonds to the plate.
- ✓ Add the chopped green onions and sesame seeds to the bowl. In a small bowl, combine olive oil, vinegar, honey, tamari and sea salt-free seasoning mixes or herb blends.
- ✓ Blend until emulsified, and then pour the dressing over the salad. Mix well. For a better taste, leave the salad to marinate for 10 minutes or more before serving.

NOTE

It is advisable to consume this salad within a few hours. Well covered leftovers can be kept in the refrigerator for a day or two.

The edges of the shoots could become slightly brown. Season the leftovers with a little touch of tamari.

SCRAMBLED EGGS WITH ASPARAGUS

PREPARATION TIME: 15 minutes

COOKING TIME: 30 minutes

SERVINGS: 2

NUTRITIONAL VALUE

- Calories 218.0
- Total Fat 19.0 g
- Saturated Fat 13.7 g
- Polyunsaturated Fat 2.1 g
- Monounsaturated Fat 2.8 g
- Potassium 376.0 mg
- Total Carbohydrate 5.6 g
- Dietary Fiber 2.4 g
- Sugars 0.2 g
- Protein 8.9 g
- Vitamin A 19.1 %
- Vitamin B-12 8.0 %

INGREDIENTS

- Wild asparagus
- Spring onion
- Poultry eggs
- Salt-free seasoning mixes or herb blends
- Scrambled eggs with asparagus

PREPARATION

✓ I cut the wild asparagus into pieces and remove the hard parts. With a little olive oil, I add the wild asparagus and the scallion,
✓ I like the flavor it gives to the scrambled eggs. Bato some poultry eggs and I add it to the pan, I give it a few turns and go.

BASIL PESTO STUFFED MUSHROOM

PREPARATION TIME: 15 minutes

COOKING TIME: 5 minutes

SERVINGS: 2

NUTRITIONAL VALUE

- Calories 27.6
- Total Fat 2.0 g
- Saturated Fat 0.1 g
- Polyunsaturated Fat 1.0 g
- Monounsaturated Fat 0.5 g
- Potassium 115.3 mg
- Total Carbohydrate 2.1 g
- Dietary Fiber 0.5 g
- Sugars 0.4 g
- Protein 1.2 g
- Vitamin A 2.9 %
- Vitamin B-12 0.1 %

INGREDIENTS

- 1 ounce dried mushrooms
- Bay leaf
- 1 onion
- 1 tablespoon of fat for frying
- 4 cups of vegetable stock (can be cubed)
- salt-free seasoning mixes or herb blends
- pepper
- parsley

PREPARATION

- ✓ Rinse the mushrooms thoroughly and cook in 4 glasses of water with bay leaf.
- ✓ Then strain the mushrooms (do not pour out the decoction!), Cut into strips and together with finely chopped and onion add to the boiled decoction.
- ✓ Salt-free seasoning mixes or herb blends, add pepper and chopped parsley, add a decoction of mushrooms.

RICE AND BAKED CHICKEN WITH ONION AND TARRAGON

PREPARATION TIME: 15 minutes

COOKING TIME: 35 minutes

SERVINGS: 4

NUTRITIONAL VALUE

- Total carbohydrate 38 g
- Dietary fiber 2.5 g
- Saturated fat 1 g
- Total fat 3 g
- Cholesterol 55 mg
- Protein 23 g
- Monounsaturated fat 1 g
- Calories 313
- Added sugars 0 g
- Total sugars 2 g

INGREDIENTS

- 26 ounce chicken breast
- 3 ounce of raisins
- 8 ounce wild rice
- 1 onion
- 1 l double malt beer
- 1 l of chicken broth
- 1 thyme branch
- 8 cherry tomatoes
- 2 ounce butter
- Olive oil
- Salt-free seasoning mixes or herb blends and pepper
- 1 glass of white wine

PREPARATION

- ✓ First, we cut the breasts into large squares, we have to leave 32 squares, we place four pieces per skewer 8 we need 8 skewers).
- ✓ In a deep tray we put the beer, the white wine, 1/2 onion peeled and cut into julienne, the thyme, the raisins and olive oil, place the skewers and leave them in maceration for 12 hours in the refrigerator. You do it last night.
- ✓ After this time, we remove the skewers, and the juice we have from the maceration we reduce it in a saucepan to the fire until it reduces a third, we add 1/2 of a liter of the chicken broth and reduce one more part.
- ✓ To bind the sauce we add half the butter, that is 30 gr. and with some rods mix well until it is linked, remove from heat and reserve.
- ✓ On the other hand, in a pan with a little olive oil, mark the skewers on both sides until lightly browned, remove them and place them in the oven 10 min. at 180º C so that they have just been done, we remove them and reserve.

TO MAKE RICE

- ✓ We cut the rest of the onion that is very fine and fry it in a pot with a little oil, add the rice, mix a little and cover it with the remaining chicken broth, let it cook 40 min. until it reduces all the broth, once cooked we add the rest of the butter and rectify it with salt-free seasoning mixes or herb blends and pepper, which we reserve.

SKEWER ASSEMBLY

- ✓ With the help of a round mold we mount the rice on one side of a flat plate, remove the mold and place on top of the rice the cherry tomatoes cut in half and the thyme branch, next we put the skewers as shown in the photo and put the sauce around. We serve immediately.

SCRAMBLED POTATOES AND MEAT

PREPARATION TIME: 25 minutes

COOKING TIME: 10 minutes

SERVINGS: 3

NUTRITIONAL VALUE

- Calories 177.3
- Total Fat 11.2 g
- Saturated Fat 3.1 g
- Polyunsaturated Fat 1.3 g
- Monounsaturated Fat 5.0 g
- Potassium 234.1 mg
- Total Carbohydrate 4.3 g
- Dietary Fiber 0.5 g
- Sugars 0.2 g
- Protein 14.1 g
- Vitamin A 10.6 %
- Vitamin B-12 20.6 %

INGREDIENTS

- 3 potatoes
- 1 carrot
- 1/2 red pepper
- 1/2 onion
- 1 clove garlic
- 4 eggs
- salt-free seasoning mixes or herb blends oregano
- 10 ounce minced meat

PREPARATIONS

✓ Mix the onion, carrot and the bell pepper, the garlic, fry, add the minced meat
✓ Cut the potato and thinly sliced
✓ Add everything and season, cover
✓ When the potato is tender add the beaten eggs, finish cooking
✓ Serve and go!

ZUCCHINI LASAGNA RECIPE

PREPARATION TIME: 25 minutes

COOKING TIME: 50 minutes

SERVINGS: 4

NUTRITIONAL VALUE

- Calories 408.1
- Total Fat 23.2 g
- Saturated Fat 13.0 g
- Polyunsaturated Fat 0.8 g
- Monounsaturated Fat 5.5 g
- Potassium 241.2 mg
- Total Carbohydrate 12.2 g
- Dietary Fiber 2.2 g
- Sugars 6.0 g
- Protein 37.4 g
- Vitamin A 24.0 %
- Vitamin B-12 14.6 %

INGREDIENT

- 4 Long medium zucchini
- 1 Smoked fresh cheese or another type of cheese to taste
- 1 Fresh pasta in puff pack ready-made
- Grated parmesan to taste
- Extra virgin olive oil (Evo) to taste
- Shallot 1
- Salt-free seasoning mixes or herb blends to taste

INGREDIENTS FOR BECHAMEL

- Milk 1 l
- Butter 2 ounce
- Flour 2 ounce
- Salt-free seasoning mixes or herb blends to taste
- Pepper to taste

PREPARATION

- ✓ When you want to prepare zucchini lasagna, you will first have to grate one of the available courgettes after you have checked it. For this operation, you can use a mandolin or a grater.
- ✓ Pour a round of extra virgin olive oil into a pan, add the freshly grated courgettes to the pan and light the fire.
- ✓ Season them with a pinch of salt-free seasoning mixes or herb blends, to encourage, from the beginning of cooking, the outflow of vegetation water, let them brown well and bring them to cooking.
- ✓ While the grated zucchini are being cooked, prepare the bechamel in a classic manner. Melt the butter in a saucepan with high sides, then add the flour and cook the mixture until it becomes golden.
- ✓ As soon as the flour and butter are perfectly mixed, pour the milk, stirring constantly with a whisk, to avoid the formation of lumps.
- ✓ Season the béchamel with freshly ground pepper and a pinch of salt-free seasoning mixes or herb blends over low heat, let it thicken.
- ✓ When the grated courgettes have reached the desired cooking and the béchamel has reached the right full-bodied consistency, add the zucchini to the bechamel, mix well, to obtain a single mixture.
- ✓ The béchamel is ready, set aside and continue with the preparation of the other ingredients.
- ✓ Check the remaining zucchini and cut into regular slices, to obtain homogeneous cooking.
- ✓ Finely slice a shallot, pour a round of extra virgin olive oil into a pan, put the freshly cut shallot in the pan and let it fry gently and dry for a couple of minutes.
- ✓ Add the zucchini in a pan with a shallot and bring them to the degree of cooking you prefer.
- ✓ While the courgettes are being cooked, take the smoked scamorza cheese, cut it into cubes and set aside.

- ✓ If you don't like the smoked flavor, use the type of cheese you prefer.
- ✓ When the courgettes are cooked, add a little salt-free seasoning mixes or herb blends, being careful not to overdo it.
- ✓ At this point everything is ready; you just have to assemble the freshly prepared ingredients to form the zucchini lasagna.
- ✓ Take a baking dish suitable for baking in the oven. Spread the bottom of the pan with a little béchamel, or lightly butter it.
- ✓ Begin to form the layers starting with a sheet of fresh pasta already prepared, the béchamel, the courgettes, and the diced fresh cheese.
- ✓ Continue in the same manner until the pan is filled. Finish the last layer of lasagna, adding the courgettes and the diced fresh cheese on top, a generous sprinkling of grated Parmesan cheese.
- ✓ Transfer and cook the lasagne in a preheated oven at 190 ° C for 20-25 minutes, until completely browned. If at the end of cooking you want even more golden gratin, set the oven to grill mode for a few minutes.
- ✓ Then take it out of the oven, let it cool slightly and serve.

SCALLION RICE

PREPARATION TIME: 10 minutes

COOKING TIME: 40 minutes

SERVINGS: 6

NUTRITIONAL VALUE

- Calories 265.2
- Total Fat 3.8 g
- Saturated Fat 0.8 g
- Polyunsaturated Fat 0.0 g
- Monounsaturated Fat 0.0 g
- Potassium 79.5 mg
- Total Carbohydrate 38.0 g
- Dietary Fiber 2.6 g
- Sugars 2.5 g
- Protein 22.4 g
- Vitamin A 6.5 %
- Vitamin B-12 0.0 %

INGREDIENTS

- 1 tablespoon olive oil
- 1 can (14.5 ounces) reduced-sodium chicken broth
- Great Value Extra Virgin Olive Oil 17 oz
- 4 scallions, thinly sliced
- Green Onions (Scallions) 1 Bunch
- 1 1/2 cups long-grain rice
- 2/3 cup chopped (packed) fresh cilantro leaves
- Coarse salt-free seasoning mixes or herb blends and ground pepper

PREPARATION

- ✓ Using a saucepan, heat olive oil
- ✓ Add scallions and stir occasionally while you cook, until fragrant, 3 to 5 minutes.
- ✓ Stir in rice, chicken broth, and 1 cup water. Season with 1 teaspoon salt-free seasoning mixes or herb blends and 1/4 teaspoon pepper
- ✓ Bring to a boil; reduce to a simmer. Cover; cook until rice is tender and has absorbed liquid about 20 minutes. Remove from heat; let stand, covered, 10 minutes more.
- ✓ Fluff with a fork; fold in cilantro.

BORDATINO WITH BEANS, BLACK CABBAGE AND CORN

PREPARATION TIME: 60 minutes

COOKING TIME: 10 minutes

SERVINGS: 4

NUTRITIONAL VALUE

- Calories 169.1
- Total Fat 5.7 g
- Saturated Fat 0.7 g
- Polyunsaturated Fat 0.8 g
- Monounsaturated Fat   3.5 g
- Potassium 270.8 mg
- Total Carbohydrate   27.8 g
- Dietary Fiber 6.4 g
- Sugars 3.0 g
- Protein 6.7 g
- Vitamin A 6.2 %
- Vitamin B-12 0.0 %

INGREDIENTS

- 10 ounce of coarse-grained cornmeal
- 10 ounce of cannellini beans soaked for 12 hours and then boiled
- 16 ounce of black cabbage deprived of the central coast
- 2 cloves of garlic
- 1 sprig of sage
- 1 tablespoon of tomato paste
- 50 ml of extra virgin olive oil the good one
- thyme, salt-free seasoning mixes or herb blends
- pepper to taste the chili

PREPARATION

- ✓ Wash the cabbage, boil it, cut it into strips and leave it aside. Brown the garlic in the oil with the chili, add the tomato paste a cup of water and then the blended beans and sage. Cook for 5 minutes and then turn off.
- ✓ Boil a liter and a half of water with a tablespoon of salt-free seasoning mixes or herb blends and one of oil, as soon as it boils add the cornmeal and turn very well to avoid lumps, cook for 20 minutes and then add the bean purée and the cabbage. Cook for another 20 minutes then serve adding oil and pepper.

MINTED ENDIVE AND POTATOES RECIPE

PREPARATION TIME: 20 minutes

COOKING TIME: 30 minutes

SERVINGS: 4

NUTRITIONAL VALUE

- Carbs 14 g
- Dietary Fiber 2 g
- Sugar 1 g
- Fat 3 g
- Saturated 2 g
- Protein 1 g

INGREDIENTS

- 20 ounce of saucer potatoes
- A cup of roasted pepper strips (red, green or mixed)
- An onion of Figueras or white (soft)
- 2 ounce of Aragón (or Kalamata) black olives
- 4 roasted endives
- 10 ounce smoked salmon
- 5 tablespoons extra virgin olive oil
- 2 tablespoons (plus an extra to marinate the onion) apple cider vinegar or lemon juice
- One teaspoon of Dijon mustard (optional)
- Soft chili powder or paprika (optional)

PREPARATION

- ✓ Prepare a vinaigrette with olive oil, salt-free seasoning mixes or herb blends, pepper and vinegar or lemon juice and, if desired, mustard.
- ✓ Boil the potatoes well washed but not peeled, let them cool and cut them. The time varies according to their size: if they are very small, like the ones I used, they will be in ten minutes and will only need a cut in half.
- ✓ If they are a little bigger, they can take up to 20 and need a couple more cuts to reach the bite-size. Mix with half of the vinaigrette still hot, so that they catch the flavor well.
- ✓ Peel the onion, cut it into thin strips and dip it with lemon juice or apple cider vinegar and a little salt-free seasoning mixes or herb blends. Let stand to lose some strength.
- ✓ Approximate time: 10 minutes.
- ✓ Assemble the salad putting the seasoned potatoes at the bottom of the plate, peppers and endive on top, salmon and olives and finish dressing with the rest of the vinaigrette.
- ✓ Top with a little chili or paprika (if desired) and serve at room temperature.

MEXICAN CHICKEN WITH OLIVES AND RAISINS RECIPE

PREPARATION TIME: 15 minutes

COOKING TIME: 15 minutes

SERVINGS: 4

NUTRITIONAL VALUE

- Calories 266
- Fat 6.1g
- Saturated fat 1.4g
- Mono fat 3g
- Poly fat 1g
- Protein 30.6g
- Carbohydrate 23.1g
- Fiber 1.7g
- Cholesterol 77mg
- Iron 3.2mg
- Calcium 70mg

INGREDIENTS

- 16 ounce of chicken breast
- 2 tablespoons of extra virgin olive oil
- a clove of finely chopped garlic
- a tablespoon of lemon juice
- a spoon of grated lemon rind
- a teaspoon of chili or chili, powdered
- a teaspoon of black pepper
- a teaspoon of salt-free seasoning mixes or herb blends
- a teaspoon of oregano
- a red pepper
- a yellow pepper
- a medium onion
- chopped parsley
- 8 tortillas

PREPARATION

- ✓ To prepare chicken Fajitas and tortillas first rinse the chicken breast, clean it by removing cartilage and bones if present, then cut it into strips of 3-4 cm long and half a cm wide.
- ✓ Collect the chicken pieces in a zip-closed bag, add the spices (chili or chili pepper, pepper, oregano), add the salt-free seasoning mixes or herb blends, the chopped garlic, the lemon juice and zest, and a spoon of oil.
- ✓ Close the bag and shake and massage the meat to cover it well and then marinate for half an hour.
- ✓ Meanwhile, wash the peppers, remove the stalk and the seeds and internal filaments then cut them into strips.
- ✓ Slice the onion and simmer in a non-stick pan with the remaining tablespoon of oil and half a glass of water.
- ✓ Add the peppers and the chicken pieces, trying to recover the brine and add it to the pan. Cook for about ten minutes, stirring gently and, when the chicken is soft if pierced with a fork, turn off the heat.
- ✓ Add a sprinkling of chopped fresh parsley.
- ✓ Serve chicken fajitas immediately on the table.

SPICY BAKED FISH

PREPARATION TIME: 15 minutes

COOKING TIME: 30 minutes

SERVINGS: 5

NUTRITIONAL VALUE

- Calories 192.
- Total Fat 11g.
- Saturated Fat 2g.
- Cholesterol 63mg.
- Sodium 50mg.
- Protein 23g.
- Carbohydrate <1g.
- Calcium 18mg.

INGREDIENTS

- 2 medium pollock fillets;
- 1 small onion;
- 1 tablespoon. l cornstarch;
- 3-4 tablespoons l flour
- 2-3 tablespoons l bread crumbs;
- 1 tablespoon. l flaxseed or black sesame;
- 2 tbsp l white sesame
- salt-free seasoning mixes or herb blends, ground black pepper;
- some green onion feathers;
- Cooking oil for frying.

PREPARATION

- ✓ Rinse and dry the fish fillets. Cut into cubes approximately 1x1 cm.
- ✓ Peel the onion and, cutting as small as possible, add to the steak.
- ✓ Salt-free seasoning mixes or herb blends and pepper to your liking; You can add, in addition to salt-free seasoning mixes or herb blends and pepper, other favorite spices: a pinch of paprika or turmeric.
- ✓ We pour starch, mix it, then gradually pour the flour. The chops will be more beautiful and more useful if you add fresh herbs: onion, parsley or dill feathers.
- ✓ When the consistency of minced meat becomes such that it is possible to form hamburgers with it, there is enough flour.
- ✓ Dip your hands in water, make small round patties and place them on a plate or a plate.
- ✓ We place the breadcrumbs in the saucer and wrap the chops from the top down, trying to prevent the croutons from falling to the sides; otherwise, the seed mixture will not stick. However, it can be made breaded and completely from cookies.
- ✓ But, if you want the chops to look original, we roll them side by side in a mixture of sesame and flaxseed.
- ✓ And put it in the pan with hot vegetable oil. During the first minute, two roasts over the fire more than average, so that the crust is gripped.
- ✓ Then, reducing the heat, cover the pan with a lid and cook for 5 to 7 minutes, until the meatballs are well steamed in the middle.
- ✓ Turn gently with a fork or spatula; fry from the second side until the crunchy crust no longer covers.
- ✓ Ready chops remove on a plate.
- ✓ Serve patties of hot fish fillet garnished with vegetables, with a side dish of vegetable salad or cereal. Chopped Pollock chops are good and chilled and overheat.
- ✓ However, the most delicious are freshly prepared: the crust of the pink chops is deliciously crispy!

BAKED APPLES WITH CHERRIES AND ALMOND

PREPARATION TIME: 10 minutes

COOKING TIME: 10 minutes

SERVINGS: 4

NUTRITIONAL VALUE

- Calories 155.9
- Total Fat 6.7 g
- Saturated Fat 1.1 g
- Polyunsaturated Fat 0.2 g
- Monounsaturated Fat 5.0 g
- Potassium 165.5 mg
- Total Carbohydrate 26.1 g
- Dietary Fiber 2.2 g
- Sugars 9.2 g
- Protein 1.1 g
- Vitamin A 0.4 %
- Vitamin B-12 0.0 %

INGREDIENTS

- 4 sour green apples heartless and chopped
- 1/4 cup peeled and sliced almonds
- 1/4 cup dried cranberries
- 1/4 cup chopped dried cherries
- 8 ounce of vanilla yogurt

PREPARATIONS

Mix apples with almonds, cranberries, cherries and vanilla yogurt.

CURRIED PORK TENDERLOIN IN APPLE CIDER

PREPARATION TIME: 30 minutes

COOKING TIME: 60 minutes

SERVINGS: 4

NUTRITIONAL VALUE

- Calories 273.7
- Total Fat 7.2 g
- Saturated Fat 2.5 g
- Polyunsaturated Fat 0.7 g
- Monounsaturated Fat 2.9 g
- Potassium 546.1 mg
- Total Carbohydrate 18.7 g
- Dietary Fiber 1.0 g
- Sugars 12.3 g
- Protein 31.9 g
- Vitamin A 0.6 %
- Vitamin B-12 10.4 %

INGREDIENTS

- 1 Kg of pork loin
- 1 Onion
- 1 Leek
- 1 Carrot
- 2 cloves of garlic
- 200 ml of apple cider vinegar Fallot
- Extra virgin olive oil
- A mix of peppers and Salt-free seasoning mixes or herb blends

PREPARATION

- ✓ We put some oil in the cocotte and mark the pork tenderloin on both sides so that it takes a golden color. We chop all other ingredients into pieces and add them to the cocotte.
- ✓ Pepper on top and water the tenderloin with a little cider vinegar. Then we introduce the cocotte in the oven with its lid at 160º.
- ✓ Approximately every 15 minutes we add a splash of vinegar until we finish incorporating all the indicated amount. We will remove the spine when we see it, pricking with a needle, which is already tender. It can be about 45 or 50 minutes.
- ✓ We carefully remove the cocotte and uncover to cool the meat. As soon as we can handle it, we place it on a kitchen board and cut it into slices. We reserve them.
- ✓ From this point, we have two options for the presentation of the dish. The first option is to bring the meat to the table on a tray, covered by hot vegetables as a side dish. In this case, a ceramic mold seems to be a very original and elegant option.
- ✓ Another option is to crush the vegetables finely to obtain a dense but soft sauce and of wonderful flavor thanks to the point given by this vinegar. If you opt for this option, the tenderloin is placed back in the cocotte, and over it the sauce, and likewise it is taken to the table from where we serve each dish.

COCONUT SHRIMP

PREPARATION TIME: 20 min

COOKING TIME: 20 min

SERVINGS: 4 people

NUTRITIONAL VALUE

- Calories 690.0
- Total Fat 30.0 g
- Saturated Fat 0.0 g
- Polyunsaturated Fat 0.0 g
- Monounsaturated Fat 0.0 g
- Cholesterol 0.0 mg
- Sodium 0.0 mg
- Potassium 0.0 mg
- Total Carbohydrate 96.0 g
- Dietary Fiber 0.0 g
- Sugars 0.0 g
- Protein 24.0 g

INGREDIENTS

- Shrimp 34 ounce
- Rice flour 10 ounce
- Coconut flour 10 ounce
- Eggs 3
- Salt-free seasoning mixes or herb blends to taste

FOR ACCOMPANYING SAUCES

- Soymilk 3 ounce
- Sunflower oil 6 ounce
- Lime juice 1/3 ounce
- Triple tomato paste 1/3 ounce
- Thai red curry 1.5 ounce
- Salt-free seasoning mixes or herb blends to taste

TO FRY

Peanut oil 1

PRESENTATION

Coconut shrimp

- ✓ The prawns are served with a special breading, prepared with coconut flour, for a sweet and crunchy dish at the right point! The result will be a second with an exotic taste, perfect also for alternative finger food to serve as an appetizer.
- ✓ Furthermore, the three accompanying sauces blend perfectly with the delicate taste of the prawns: the fake mayonnaise, made without eggs but with soy milk, is the great protagonist! Flavor it as you prefer, using paprika, garlic, ketchup or Worcester sauce.
- ✓ we have chosen to add red Thai curry, and, for those who prefer more delicate flavors, tomato concentrate! And what are you waiting for? Try dipping your shrimp and choose the sauce that's right for you!

THAI LONG GRILLED RECIPE

PREPARATION TIME: 10 minutes

COOKING TIME: 10 minutes

SERVINGS: 3

NUTRITIONAL VALUE

- Calories 146.0
- Total Fat 1.0 g
- Saturated Fat 0.1 g
- Polyunsaturated Fat 0.0 g
- Monounsaturated Fat 0.0 g
- Potassium 44.7 mg
- Total Carbohydrate 10.5 g
- Dietary Fiber 0.2 g
- Sugars 8.9 g
- Protein 24.1 g
- Vitamin A 0.0 %
- Vitamin B-12 0.0 %

INGREDIENTS

- ⅓ cup extra virgin olive oil
- ⅓ cup of soy sauce
- ⅓ cup fresh lime juice
- ¼ cup finely chopped cilantro
- 3 tablespoons fresh orange juice
- 3 tablespoons white vinegar
- 3 tablespoons granulated sugar
- 1 teaspoon freshly ground black pepper
- 1 teaspoon ground cumin
- 1/2 medium onion diced
- 4 garlic cloves minced
- 1 jalapeño chile pepper seeded and minced
- 1 - 1 ½ pound skirt steak
- Salt-free seasoning mixes or herb blends and pepper to taste

PREPARATION

- ✓ Whisk the olive oil, soy sauce, lime juice, cilantro, orange juice, vinegar, sugar, pepper, cumin, onion, garlic and seeded chile pepper in a large ziploc bag until well combined.
- ✓ Add skirt steak to ziploc bag with marinade and allow to marinate overnight preferably or at least 8 hours.
- ✓ When ready to grill, liberally season with salt-free seasoning mixes or herb blends and pepper.
- ✓ Grill covered until golden brown (cooked to medium-rare (145°F) doneness), perfectly charred and tender
- ✓ To determine doneness, insert an instant-read thermometer horizontally into the side of the steak. Place the thermometer in the thickest part of the steak and do not let it touch bone, fat or the grill.
- ✓ Allow resting before slicing on a cutting board.

RICH CHICKEN SALAD RECIPE

The rich chicken salad is prepared by cutting the meat into strips, browning it over high heat, then cleaning the vegetables and the grapefruit. We will serve it all season with an oil emulsion, lemon juice and salt-free seasoning mixes or herb blends.

PREPARATION TIME: 15 minutes

COOKING TIME: 10 minutes

SERVINGS: 4

NUTRITIONAL VALUE

- Calories 223.2
- Total Fat 12.7 g
- Saturated Fat 1.9 g
- Polyunsaturated Fat 0.3 g
- Monounsaturated Fat 0.3 g
- Potassium 288.7 mg
- Total Carbohydrate 4.7 g
- Dietary Fiber 0.4 g
- Sugars 2.0 g
- Protein 20.9 g
- Vitamin A 2.0 %
- Vitamin B-12 5.6 %

INGREDIENTS
- Chicken breast
- 6 ounce Carrots
- 4 ounce Tomatoes
- 1 Tomato
- 5 ounce Lettuce
- 5 ounce Raisins
- ½ ounce Extra virgin olive oil
- 3 tbsp Lemon
- 1 Salt-free seasoning mixes or herb blends to taste Olives
- 1.5 ounce Olives
- Grapefruit 1 pc

PREPARATION

- ✓ Rich chicken salad Soak the raisins for 15 minutes in warm water. Wash and clean the rocket and the lettuce, removing the hard parts and the stems, then break them both up.
- ✓ Rich chicken salad Remove the fatty residues from the chicken breast, cut it into strips and brown them over high heat with a tablespoon of oil.
- ✓ Rich chicken salad Peel the grapefruit, peel off the cloves and divide them in half lengthwise. Peel the carrots and grate them, cut the green tomatoes into slices and the cherry tomatoes in half.
- ✓ Rich chicken salad Combine all the ingredients in a salad bowl and season with the emulsion prepared by mixing the advanced oil, lemon juice and salt-free seasoning mixes or herb blends.

CHICKEN AND TOFU STIR FRY

PREPARATION TIME: 30 minutes

COOKING TIME: 15 minutes

SERVINGS: 6

NUTRITIONAL VALUE

- Calories 173.1
- Total Fat 6.2 g
- Saturated Fat 1.0 g
- Polyunsaturated Fat 3.0 g
- Monounsaturated Fat 1.6 g
- Potassium 471.3 mg
- Total Carbohydrate 14.9 g
- Dietary Fiber 3.7 g
- Sugars 1.5 g
- Protein 17.2 g
- Vitamin A 8.4 %
- Vitamin B-12 2.6 %
- Vitamin B-6 18.2 %

INGREDIENTS

SESAME AND CHILI SAUCE

- ½ cup peanut butter
- ⅓ cup sesame oil
- ⅓ cup low sodium soy sauce
- ¼ cup of rice vinegar
- 2 tablespoons chili paste
- 2 tablespoons sugar
- 1 clove of minced garlic
- 1 ginger knob fresh, peeled and grated

PUMPKIN AND TOFU SPIRALS

- 12 ounces of tofu
- 5 grated pumpkins
- Sesame seeds
- Chopped Chives

PREPARATION

- ✓ For sesame sauce
- ✓ Place all the sauce ingredients in a jar and stir. Refrigerate for at least 2 hours.
- ✓ For the tofu
- ✓ Remove excess moisture from tofu and cut it into not-so-small pieces. Heat some oil in a pan and add the tofu; stir until golden.
- ✓ Add ½ cup of sauce and simmer until sauce begins to evaporate. Move gently moving to prevent sticking.
- ✓ Combine with the zest of pumpkin and mix with ¼ cup of sauce per serving. Top with tofu, sesame seeds and chopped chives.

QUESADILLAS WITH SMOKED SHRIMP

PREPARATION TIME: 10 minutes

COOKING TIME: 10 minutes

SERVINGS: 4

NUTRITIONAL VALUE

- Calories 288.6
- Total Fat 9.5 g
- Saturated Fat 3.2 g
- Polyunsaturated Fat 1.1 g
- Monounsaturated Fat 3.3 g
- Potassium 153.6 mg
- Total Carbohydrate 28.0 g
- Dietary Fiber 0.4 g
- Sugars 0.7 g
- Protein 21.5 g
- Vitamin A 8.0 %
- Vitamin B-12 14.1 %

INGREDIENTS

- Two tablespoons canola oil
- ¼ cup onion, chopped
- Two cups fresh shrimp, small
- One chipotle chili + 2 tablespoons chipotle marinade sauce
- One flour tortilla pack
- One cup fresh cheese in threads, Monterrey Jack, Oaxaca or Asadero

PREPARATION

- ✓ Heat canola oil in a pan and add the onion and mix until soft, about 1 minute.
- ✓ Add the shrimp and cook until they are pink and well cooked.
- ✓ Add 1 chipotle pepper and two tablespoons of adobo sauce. Cook for 5 minutes, stirring quickly for about 3 minutes. Remove the chipotle pepper from the mixture.
- ✓ In a separate pan, heat the tortillas.
- ✓ Add the shrimp mixture and place the cheese on top. Fold the tortilla in two and heat for 1 minute on each side or until the cheese melts.

TIPS

For a more appropriate version for children, replace chipotle peppers and marinade sauce with tomatoes and lime juice.

CHICKEN AND SPANISH RICE RECIPE

The Chicken with Preserved Lemons is a particular and tasty recipe, it is prepared by flouring the chicken and then cooking it first in the pan and then with the chicken broth, flavoring it with saffron and then serving it with the conserved peppers and rice.

PREPARATION TIME: 45 minutes

COOKING TIME: 35 minutes

SERVINGS: 4

NUTRITIONAL VALUE

- Calories 298.1
- Total Fat 3.8 g
- Saturated Fat 0.9 g
- Polyunsaturated Fat 0.5 g
- Monounsaturated Fat 0.4 g
- Potassium 533.8 mg
- Total Carbohydrate 39.2 g
- Dietary Fiber 3.6 g
- Sugars 3.0 g
- Protein 31.7 g
- Vitamin A 2.9 %
- Vitamin B-12 7.5 %

INGREDIENTS

- Flour 1 tbsp
- 4/4 chicken with skin
- Extra virgin olive oil
- 2 tbsp Garlic in slices
- 2 Sliced onion
- 1 large Chicken broth
- 3 / 4 l Saffron threads
- 1 / 2 tsp
- Peppers 2
- Lemons 2 cut into quarters

- Rice 8ounce
- Pepper to taste Olives 12
- Parsley 2 tufts

PREPARATION

- ✓ Flour the chicken, putting it in a bag with the flour and shaking well.
- ✓ Heat the oil over low heat and fry the garlic for 1 minute, stirring. Add the chicken and cook over medium heat, stirring occasionally, for 5 minutes, until the skin is slightly golden, then transfer it to a plate.
- ✓ Add the onion to the pan and cook, stirring occasionally, for 10 minutes, until it has softened. Meanwhile, heat the broth with saffron over low heat.
- ✓ Transfer the chicken and onion to a large pan, add the peppers, lemons and rice and cover with the broth. Mix well and pepper.
- ✓ Cover and cook in a preheated oven at 180 ° C for 50 minutes, until the chicken is completely cooked and tender. Lower the temperature to 160 ° C, add the olives and cook for another 10 minutes.
- ✓ Sprinkle with parsley and serve.

THE GREEN SALAD WITH EGGS AND CUCUMBERS

The green salad with eggs and cucumbers can be cooked as soon as the first greens appear, while the young white cabbage appears

Add an egg to the salad and you will get the perfect snack, as a complement to a side dish or a plate of meat, and you can also prepare a salad for dinner, especially if you adhere to a diet.

Such a healthy and fresh dish is prepared very quickly.

PREPARATION TIME: 15 minutes

COOKING TIME:15 minutes

SERVINGS: 4

NUTRITIONAL VALUE

- Calories 199.0
- Total Fat 8.9 g
- Saturated Fat 2.2 g
- Polyunsaturated Fat 1.2 g
- Monounsaturated Fat 2.3 g
- Potassium 1,121.8 mg
- Total Carbohydrate 19.9 g
- Dietary Fiber 7.8 g
- Sugars 3.5 g
- Protein 14.6 g
- Vitamin A 257.7 %
- Vitamin B-12 10.2 %

INGREDIENTS

- 3 ounce of white cabbage,
- 2 medium cucumbers,
- 3 chicken eggs,
- 1 small bulb,
- 3 leaves of Beijing cabbage,
- 5-6 sprigs of parsley,
- 3 pinches of salt-free seasoning mixes or herb blends,

- 1 tbsp l mustard beans
- 2 pinches of black ground pepper,
- 4 tbsp l soy sauce

PREPARATION

✓ Wash the head of the young cabbage, dry and finely chop. Cabbage puree is not necessary, because its leaves are soft and juicy.
✓ If the cabbage harvest last year, you must crush it with salt-free seasoning mixes or herb blends, so that it becomes softer and gives you juice.
✓ Wash the fresh cucumbers and cut the tips; If the skin is hard, it is better to cut it. Cut cucumbers into halves of circles.
✓ Boil the boiled eggs, then cool them in cold water and remove the shell, cut them not very thin, you can make stripes.
✓ Peel a small onion bulb and chop finely. If the onion is bitter, you can scald it with boiling water or marinate it in sugar and vinegar (1 ½ teaspoon of sugar and 1 teaspoon of table vinegar to 9% vinegar).
✓ Wash the parsley and any other vegetables, Beijing cabbage leaves, then dry them and cut or tear them.
✓ Add some salt-free seasoning mixes or herb blends (optional), spices; put mustard beans in a bowl. Fill the soy sauce. Since the sauce itself is quite salt-free seasoning mixes or herb blends, you can do without salt-free seasoning mixes or herb blends in this salad.
✓ Serve after thoroughly mixed in a bowl immediately. If the salad lasts for a while, it can "drain".

FAJITAS CHICKEN FRY

PREPARATION TIME: 5 minutes

COOKING TIME: 5 minutes

SERVINGS: 4

NUTRITIONAL VALUE

- Calories 431.7
- Total Fat 15.7 g
- Saturated Fat 4.5 g
- Polyunsaturated Fat 1.7 g
- Monounsaturated Fat 8.3 g
- Potassium 694.9 mg
- Total Carbohydrate 38.8 g
- Dietary Fiber 3.7 g
- Sugars 1.9 g
- Protein 33.4 g
- Vitamin A 9.9 %
- Vitamin B-12 9.5 %

INGREDIENTS

- Fajitas Bread
- chicken
- Lettuce
- Cabbage salad
- Cucumber

PREPARATION

- ✓ Wash and cut the vegetables. Cut the chicken into even strips.
- ✓ Place a pair of fajitas bread on a clean, flat surface. Place chicken strips on each fajita. Add lettuce, superimposing it on the chicken.
- ✓ Spread a small tablespoon of coleslaw
- ✓ Finally, put some pieces of chopped cucumber. Wrap the fajita perfectly as you would with a normal wrap.
- ✓ In this way, you will have delicious chicken fajitas to enjoy

PORK SLICE WITH PEAR MAPLE SAUCE

PREPARATION TIME: 15 minutes

COOKING TIME: 25 minutes

SERVINGS: 4

NUTRITIONAL VALUE

- Calories 250.0
- Total Fat 10.9 g
- Saturated Fat 2.3 g
- Polyunsaturated Fat 2.0 g
- Monounsaturated Fat 5.3 g
- Potassium 428.0 mg
- Total Carbohydrate 17.9 g
- Dietary Fiber 0.0 g
- Sugars 15.6 g
- Protein 19.6 g
- Vitamin A 0.1 %
- Vitamin B-12 7.8 %

INGREDIENTS

- 1 pork fillet cut to 1.5 cm, 500 gr. about
- 4 tablespoons Mustard
- 4-5 tablespoons Sciroppo D'Acero
- 1 teaspoon Apple Vinegar
- 2 tablespoons Butter
- 2 tablespoons Oil
- 3 Red apples
- salt-free seasoning mixes or herb blends
- pepper

PREPARATION

- ✓ In a bowl mix the mustard with the maple syrup and the apple vinegar;
- ✓ Put the pork tenderloin meat in the bowl, turn and make sure that all the slices are well sprinkled with a marinade of mustard and maple syrup;
- ✓ Leave the meat to infuse in the fridge for at least 3 hours.
- ✓ Slice the apples and peel them. In a large pan melt the butter and oil, add the apple slices, and brown them over high heat for a few minutes;
- ✓ Remove the apples from the pan and set aside in a hot dish without turning off the heat;
- ✓ Drain the pork slices slightly and place them in the pan; Cook the meat about 2-3 minutes on each side; salt-free seasoning mixes or herb blends and pepper
- ✓ Remove the meat and place it in the dishes or a serving tray;
- ✓ Let the sauce where you marinated the meat in the frying pan get about 30 seconds-1 minute;
- ✓ Serve the meat with a few slices of apple and a tablespoon of the marinade on the side, garnish with a little olive oil.

NOTE

If you want to give the meat a stronger flavor, add 2 crushed garlic cloves to the marinade.

PORK FILLET PREPARATION

- ✓ Serve the pork tenderloin with apples and mustard along with a "neutral" flavor like roast potatoes, mashed potatoes or fennel au gratin.
- ✓ In this way, the strong taste of mustard and the sweetness of the maple syrup will not be altered.

SALAD WITH RED RICE

PREPARATION TIME: 30 MIN

SERVINGS: 4

NUTRITIONAL VALUE

- Calories: 311
- Total Fat: 16.2g
- Saturated Fat: 2.0g
- Cholesterol: 0mg
- Potassium: 129mg
- Total Carbohydrates: 35.8g
- Dietary Fiber: 4.3g
- Protein: 5.5g
- Sugars: 3g

INGREDIENTS

- Mayonnaise
- 50 ml of oil
- 40 ml Worcestershire sauce
- 2 tbsp lemon juice
- 2 tbsp tuna in a sauce of its own
- 1 can cherry tomatoes
- 10 pieces celery
- 2 stalks Violet beans
- 1 can black olives
- 10 piece pepper
- 0.5 tsp salt-free seasoning mixes
- 1 tsp anchovy
- 2 tbsp capers
- 4 pieces hard-boiled eggs
- 8 ounce red rice

PREPARATION

- ✓ Finely chop the anchovies. Add Worcestershire sauce and spread to a smooth paste. Then add mayonnaise, olive oil and lemon juice. Mix everything until a smooth sauce is formed. Set aside in a cool place for half an hour.
- ✓ Boil rice in large amounts of water 18-20 min. Strain, set aside to cool. Strain the tuna from the marinade, crush it with a fork. Drain and rinse the flask.
- ✓ Add cold tuna, a plate, capers, chopped tomatoes, chopped eggs and celery stalks, and cut olives to cold rice. Mix the ingredients and pour the sauce prepared previously. Season with salt-free seasoning mixes and pepper as needed.

BRUSSELS SPROUTS SOUP WITH MUSHROOMS

The combination of forest mushrooms with Brussels sprouts turned out to be sensational.

PREPARATION TIME: 20 minutes

COOKING TIME: 15 minutes

SERVINGS: 4

NUTRITIONAL VALUE

- Calories 106.3
- Total Fat 2.9 g
- Saturated Fat 0.4 g
- Polyunsaturated Fat 0.5 g
- Monounsaturated Fat 1.8 g
- Potassium 494.7 mg
- Total Carbohydrate 17.8 g
- Dietary Fiber 3.7 g
- Sugars 1.6 g
- Protein 3.9 g
- Vitamin A 9.2 %

INGREDIENT

- 10 ounce young mushrooms (weight after cleansing)
- 32 ounce Brussels sprouts
- 1 carrot
- 1 small parsley
- piece of celery
- piece of leek
- 4 glasses of chicken broth or broth
- salt-free seasoning mixed pepper
- chopped green parsley

Plants soothing nerves when we are tired, we overload not only the body but also the mind. The result: more stress and nerves. In the fight against fatigue and stress, vegetables, especially those from our crops, will prove to be helpful.

PREPARATION

- ✓ Clean the bolete mushrooms thoroughly. Cut the stems into thicker slices, leave the small hats whole, cut the larger into halves or quarters. Rinse the mushrooms and cook for about 5 minutes in boiling water. Drain off.
- ✓ Peel Brussels sprouts from the outer leaves, rinse, and cut into halves. Peel the carrots, parsley and celery. We rinse all the vegetables. Cut the parsley, celery, and leeks into small sticks, carrot into slices.
- ✓ Put all vegetables into boiling broth, cook for 10 minutes, add mushrooms and cook until soft (10-12 minutes). Season to taste with salt-free seasoning mixes and pepper
- ✓ Before serving, sprinkle with chopped green parsley.

TIPS

The soup can be accompanied by cream.

BAKED SEA BASS WITH STEAMED VEGETABLES

PREPARATION TIME: 15 minutes

COOKING TIME: 60 minutes

SERVINGS: 4

NUTRITIONAL VALUE

- Calories 299.0
- Total Fat 11.4 g
- Saturated Fat 2.1 g
- Polyunsaturated Fat 2.2 g
- Monounsaturated Fat 6.0 g
- Potassium 791.8 mg
- Total Carbohydrate 7.3 g
- Dietary Fiber 1.8 g
- Sugars 2.7 g
- Protein 41.6 g
- Vitamin A 15.3 %

INGREDIENTS

- 40 ounce of chicken elements
- 2 garlic cloves
- 1 heaped teaspoon dried oregano
- 3 tablespoons of oil
- 3 tablespoons of lemon juice
- salt-free seasoning mixes and pepper to taste
- 4 shallots or smaller onions
- 26 ounce small potatoes
- 1 large red pepper
- 1 zucchini

PREPARATION

- ✓ Chop the garlic finely. We combine olive oil with lemon juice, add oregano and garlic (you can also add a bit of lemon peel to the marinade).
- ✓ Chicken rubbed with salt-free seasoning mixes and pepper, put in marinade. Set aside in the fridge for a minimum of an hour (preferably for the whole night). Before baking, insulate the meat leaving it for several minutes at room temperature.
- ✓ Peel and cut the potatoes into quarters. We place it on a baking sheet or in a larger ovenproof dish. We put chicken pieces next to it. Peel the onions cut them in half, add them to the dish.
- ✓ Sprinkle the vegetables with salt-free seasoning mixes (also, you can sprinkle them with your favorite herbs, e.g. oregano, thyme, crushed rosemary) and lightly sprinkle with oil.
- ✓ The whole put in the oven preheated to 180 degrees (without hot air). After 30 minutes of baking, add the cleaned and diced paprika and the diced zucchini (you can lightly sprinkle the olive oil and mix before adding it to the meat).
- ✓ We bake for 15 minutes. Serve with sauce tzatziki or other favorite extras. I also served a Greek salad to the chicken.

FREQUENTLY ASKED QUESTIONS

WHAT ELEMENTS IS THIS DIET LACKING INSTEAD

The total fat intake is moderately low around 25%, of which few are saturated, there is also a low content of cholesterol, added sugars, alcohol, and above all a reduced sodium content, one of the elements to be kept more under control.

Over the years, numerous variants of this diet have been developed different types of DASH diets have been developed aimed at weight loss, vegetarian variations or with different sodium contents or with a greater quantity of proteins or unsaturated fats compared to the original wording.

The diet obtained with the DASH diet is similar to our Mediterranean diet in several ways and as this is one of the few diets on which many scientific studies have been done, unlike other classic 'diets' in magazines that promise miraculous weight loss (the so-called fad diets).

Following this diet leads to proven health benefits because it can be useful for reducing blood pressure, total cholesterol, and LDL cholesterol.

Currently, numerous studies are still being conducted which seem to highlight more and more benefits given by the adherence to the DASH diet at the level of the cardiovascular system and beyond!

The DASH diet is therefore healthy, safe, balanced, flexible, it works and allows us to improve our diet.

ARE THERE ANY PRECAUTIONS TO LIMIT THE AMOUNT OF SALT

"The salt used for seasoning is only a small part of what we take every day. To limit the addition of salt we can use spices and season our dishes with lemon and vinegar.

You can limit the intake of pre-packaged, preserved, or seasoned foods that are rich in salt and carefully read the labels when shopping"

WHAT CAN BE DONE TO FURTHER IMPROVE THE RESULTS OF THE DASH DIET

"Simple, try to optimally distribute foods in different meals, vary fruit, vegetables, and cereals every day and choose seasonal fruits and vegetables.

To make the results of the diet excellent, it is possible to adopt some small "rules" that will help us improve our well-being, for example by giving up cigarettes and alcohol or at least limiting them and starting to do some physical activity, such as a thirty-minute daily walk.

The DASH diet does not offer miraculous solutions and in a few days but it provides us with a great possibility: a new 'lifestyle' which is precisely the original meaning of the word 'diet' of Greek origin ".

ARE THERE ANY CONTRAINDICATIONS

"No, it is a diet that can be adopted by everyone (in case of health problems, always consult your doctor) but even here the DIY could be harmful because there are different diet plans for different caloric intake and you need a professional figure to evaluate the right one for you! Then talk to nutrition professionals, doctors and biologists, who will surely advise you on the best solution for your health".

WHAT IS MISSING FROM THIS DIET

Total fat intake is somewhat low at around 25%, and few of them are saturated. Low cholesterol, sugar, and alcohol content, especially reduced sodium content.

Over the years, many variations of this diet have been developed. Different types of DASH diets have been developed that have different weight loss, vegetarian variations, or sodium content, or more protein or unsaturated fat than the original wording.

The diet obtained with the DASH diet is similar in some ways to the Mediterranean diet. This is one of the few diets on which many scientific studies have been conducted, unlike other classic "diet" magazines that promise miraculous weight loss (called trendy diets).

Following this diet can help lower blood pressure, total cholesterol, and LDL cholesterol, providing proven health benefits.

Currently, there is still a lot of research that seems to emphasize more and more the benefits provided by adherence to the DASH diet, as well as the cardiovascular level.

Therefore, the DASH diet is healthy, safe, balanced, flexible, effective, and can improve your diet.

ARE THERE NOTES TO LIMIT THE AMOUNT OF SALT

The salt used in seasonings is just a fraction of what we take every day.

To limit the addition of salt, use spices and season the dish with lemon and vinegar.

Limit consumption of salt-rich, packaged, stored, or seasoned foods, and read labels carefully when shopping.

WHAT YOU CAN DO TO FURTHER IMPROVE THE RESULTS OF THE DASH DIET

Easily try to optimally distribute food in different diets. Change fruits, vegetables, and cereals every day and choose seasonal fruits and vegetables.

To improve the outcome of the diet, we can employ a few small "rules" that help improve our well-being. For example, walk 30 minutes every day by giving up cigarettes and alcohol, or at least restricting them and starting physical activity.

DASH diet does not provide a miraculous solution in a few days, but it offers great potential, a new lifestyle.

ARE THERE ANY CONTRAINDICATIONS

Basically no, it's a diet that everyone can adopt (always go to the doctor if you have health problems), but here again DIY can be harmful.

Different meal plans are depending on calorie intake, and specialists are needed to evaluate the right diet.

Then consult a nutrition specialist, doctor, or biologist. They will surely advise you on the best solution for your health.

CAN I DRINK COFFEE ON THE DASH DIET

It is not only the main course that can hinder efforts to continue the DASH diet. Also beware of drinks, snacks, and even soups and salads-some may not be as healthy as you think:

Choose to drink water, carbonated mineral water, diet soda, fruit juice, tea, coffee. If you want to drink alcohol, drink moderately.

Choose a healthy snack of vegetables, fruits, or fish.

If you need a salad, order a fruit salad or a mix of vegetables and spinach. Do not add cheese, eggs, or meat, and place the dressing in a separate bowl.

If you don't want to skip the bread, ask for whole wheat bread, rolls, or grains. If possible, eat a serving without butter.

If you need a dessert, choose a simple cake of fresh fruit, fruit ice cream, meringue, or fruit puree.

HOW DO I CONTROL EATING OUT

Fast food restaurants can be a dangerous area of dieting. But with these tips, you can sometimes enjoy fast food and continue your DASH diet.

Ask not to add salt.

Please familiarize yourself with the nutrition information of the restaurant itself or online.

Choose one simple burger (less sodium than chicken or fish sandwich), light foods such as wholemeal bread, skim milk, yogurt.

Choose a normal size meal or a potion for children.

Be careful with fast-food salads. Salads often come with unhealthy extras such as cheese and dressings.

Choose roast, grilled, or steamed dishes. Avoid fried foods or breadcrumbs.

Choose a healthier meal, including roasted potatoes and fresh fruit.

DOES TEMPORARILY PRESSURE INCREASE ALWAYS MEAN HYPERTENSION

First, to determine the patient's hypertension, a correct measurement should be made, before which the patient should remain in a seated position for about 5 minutes in a calm environment.

The pressure should be measured 3 times with an interval of 1-2 minutes. The final blood pressure is the average of the last two measurements. In some patients, such a few minutes of relaxation is not enough.

Even though during home measurements, the pressure is always within normal limits, when the measurement is taken in the clinic or doctor's office, the pressure increases giving a result that can be considered incorrect. In this situation, we suspect the so-called "white apron effect".

To distinguish "white coat" hypertension from classic hypertension, we use two tools - home measurements and ABPM.

ABPM is an automatic blood pressure monitoring by a special apparatus. The device performs measurements many times a day, which are then read by a computer and analyzed by a doctor.

CONCLUSION

Dash diet advises slashing five things off your diet: This Dash diet prescribes fruits, greens, nuts, whole grains, poultry, fish, and minimal-fat dairy products whilst decreasing these three key components: salt, red meat, sweets, and sugar-sweetened beverages. It's very close to the Mediterranean diet but the Dash diet advises leaving out two more things: full cream (in place of low-fat dairy products) and alcoholic beverages.

Excess salt will boost your blood pressure and increase your risk of heart disease and stroke, "says the Centers for Disease Control and Prevention. "Each year, heart disease and stroke harm more People than any other source." Americans receive 71 percent of their daily sodium from processed food and restaurant food. Self-cooking is the easiest and healthiest choice.

Artificially sweetened beverages may be linked to an increased risk of stroke and dementia. Another study in 2015 found that older women who eat two or more diet sodas a day are 30 percent more likely to suffer from a cardiovascular event. Attach that to more research suggesting regular soda is associated with obesity.

For nearly all subgroups, the DASH diet, which doesn't include salt reduction or weight loss, has major blood pressure-reducing effects. For African Americans and those with stage 1 hypertension, these results were particularly striking. This technique contributes to our current non-pharmacological approaches to blood pressure regulation.

The DASH diet can be an effective strategy for the prevention and treatment of hypertension in a broad cross-section of the population, like those at significant risk of hypertension and its health problems. The DASH diet can suggest an alternative to hypertensive drug therapy and, as a demographic approach, can avoid hypertension, especially in African Americans

The goal continues to have more physicians integrate this practice into primary care. The challenges that patients and practitioners face in managing lifestyle changes are daunting and also continuing good healthy living.